Sometimes You Just Want to Feel Like a Human Being

This book is printed on recycled paper. ♻

Sometimes You Just Want to Feel Like a Human Being

Case Studies of Empowering Psychotherapy with People with Disabilities

by

Mary Ann Blotzer, L.C.S.W.-C.

and

Richard Ruth, Ph.D.

with invited contributors

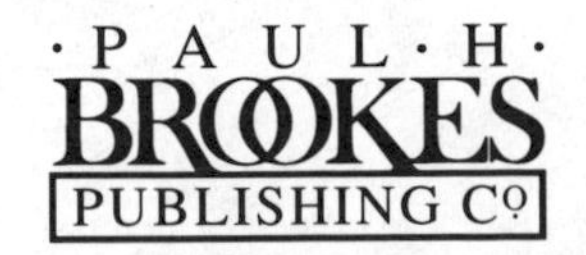

Baltimore • London • Toronto • Sydney

Paul H. Brookes Publishing Co.
Post Office Box 10624
Baltimore, Maryland 21285-0624

Typeset by Brushwood Graphics, Inc., Baltimore, Maryland.
Manufactured in the United States of America by
The Maple Press Company, York, Pennsylvania.

Names of clients in this book are pseudonyms. Identifying information has been altered to protect privacy.

Mary Ann Blotzer and Richard Ruth have shared equally the writing and editing tasks involved in the chapters they have co-authored and the assembling of this book. Their names are listed in alphabetical order.

Library of Congress Cataloging-in-Publication Data

Sometimes you just want to feel like a human being: case studies of empowering psychotherapy with people with disabilities / by Mary Ann Blotzer and Richard Ruth.
p. cm.
Includes bibliographical references and index.
ISBN 1-55766-196-0
1. Handicapped—Mental health—Case studies. 2. Psychotherapy—Case studies. 3. Handicapped—Rehabilitation—Case studies. I. Blotzer, Mary Ann. II. Ruth, Richard.
RC451.4.H35S66 1996
616.89'14—dc20
95-11590
CIP

British Library Cataloguing-in-Publication data are available from the British Library.

Contents

Contributors

THE AUTHORS

Mary Ann Blotzer, L.C.S.W.-C., is a clinical social worker and disability rights advocate in private practice in Wheaton, Maryland. She specializes in the areas of disability, chronic illness, and Alzheimer's disease. Formerly the director of the Developmental Disabilities Program at Community Psychiatric Clinic, she is currently affiliated with the Arc of Montgomery County and with the Health and Human Services Department of Montgomery County. She is a fellow of the American Orthopsychiatric Association.

Richard Ruth, Ph.D., is trained as a psychologist, a neuropsychologist, a psychoanalyst, and a family therapist. He is bilingual in Spanish and bicultural. Currently he is in private practice in Wheaton, Maryland; serves as Acting Chief Psychologist at Community Psychiatric Clinic in Montgomery County, Maryland; is a member of the faculty of Trinity College, Washington, D.C., and the University of Virginia, Falls Church, Virginia; and is Director of the Puerto Rico Research Institute, Washington, D.C. He is the chair of the Study Group on Disability of the American Orthopsychiatric Association.

THE CONTRIBUTORS

Donald Cassidy, Ph.D., is a licensed psychologist and educator. He currently serves as Head of School for Fox Valley School in Montgomery County, Maryland. He is a former director of the Developmental Disabilities Program of Community Psychiatric Clinic, where he was also a staff psychologist. Dr. Cassidy has 10 years' experience as an educator in small Quaker schools. A graduate of Swarthmore College and The Fielding Institute, he received training in American Sign Language at Gallaudet College.

Karen Donovan, L.C.S.W., is a clinical social worker in private practice in Los Angeles. She has been practicing psychotherapy for over 14 years, specializing in work with people with disabilities. She is a clinical associate in the Los Angeles Institute and Society For Psychoanalytic Studies. She consults with the mental health community on issues related to disability.

Paul B. Feuerstein, C.S.W., has been Executive Director of Barrier Free Living in New York City since 1981. Prior to that, he was Associate Director of Project

Outward Bound, a research project with people with new disabilities that led to the development of Barrier Free Living. He has a master's of social work from Hunter School of Social Work, a master's of sacred theology from General Theological Seminary and a master's of art from New York University School of Education. He was founder and first chairperson of a Citywide Coalition on Housing for People with Disabilities and was chairperson of the Diocese of New York's Commission on Ministry with Persons with Disabilities.

JoAnn LeMaistre, Ph.D., is a clincial assistant professor in the department of psychiatry and the behavioral sciences, Stanford University School of Medicine. She is a psychologist in full-time private practice. She lectures widely on psychological sequalae of medical illness/disability and participates in the training of psychiatry residents and postdoctoral psychology interns at Stanford. She is the author of *Beyond Rage: Mastering Unavoidable Health Changes;* a companion audiotape; and *Frank Talk,* a video about the emotional complexities of disabling illness.

Adele Natter, L.C.S.W.-C., is a psychiatric social worker who has been employed at Community Psychiatric Clinic in Montgomery County, Maryland, since 1983. For the past several years, she has worked in the Developmental Disabilities Program, helping to develop mental health options for persons with developmental disabilities.

Rhoda Olkin, Ph.D., is an associate professor of psychology at the California School of Professional Psychology, where she is also the adviser to students with disabilities. She has a clinical practice and consultation service in Walnut Creek, California.

Jean Finkelstein Ratner, L.C.S.W., is a graduate of Smith College and holds a master's degree in clinical social work from Simmons School of Social Work. She was the chief social worker of West-Ros-Park Mental Health Center in Boston. Now based in Washington, D.C., and Montgomery County, Maryland, she is a consultant at Community Psychiatric Clinic. In her private practice she treats anxiety and depression in adults. She has begun specializing in cognitive-behavioral therapy as well as psychodynamically oriented therapy.

Ann Steiner, Ph.D., M.F.C.C., practices psychotherapy in the San Francisco Bay Area. She is an assistant clinical professor in the department of psychiatry, University of California Medical School in San Francisco; a fellow of the American Group Psychotherapy Association; and a former president of the Northern California Group Psychotherapy Society. Dr. Steiner specializes in individual and group therapy with adults dealing with medical illness, trauma, and relationship issues. Her personal experience with chronic illness has enhanced her awareness of the need for flexibility and creativity in treatment.

Foreword

> It was once said that the moral test of government is how that government treats those who are in the dawn of life, the children; those who are in the twilight of life, the elderly; and those who are in the shadows of life—the sick, the needy, and the handicapped. (Senator Hubert Humphrey, November 1, 1977)

Two powerful conflicting attitudes toward people with disabilities have permeated U.S. social history: callousness and compassion. These two attitudes were typified in a recent event. A friend of mine, whose legs are paralyzed, was traveling on a well-known airline. He was accommodated in the airport with the required wheelchair, accompanied by airport personnel who were very sensitive to his needs. Once he was in the process of actually boarding the plane in his wheelchair, however, one employee blurted out loudly and angrily, "Why don't you just get up and walk to your seat!"

The callousness toward those who have disabilities reflected in that remark may have personal origins. Nevertheless, it also reflects the Social Darwinism that pervades the American experience, a view that has often been tied to the historical survival struggle of the expansion of the West. This callous attitude is being perpetuated to the present day by three values underlying the social structure of the United States: power, perfection, and productivity.

Power In American culture, disability has historically been tied to weakness. One need only remember the extraordinary efforts that were made to hide President Roosevelt's paralysis, lest the image be conveyed that he was not a strong leader. Disability continues to be associated with impotence, pervasive intellectual and social limitations, and the inability to stand up for one's principles.

Perfection The popularity of cosmetic surgery in the United States testifies to the strong wish for the body perfect. Combined with the optimism implicit in the American belief that anything can be fixed, changes are made to reach an ideal standard of beauty and perfection both in appearance and in thought. Any disability is seen as an imperfection and is therefore a threat to one's self-image.

Productivity U.S. society has been built on individual productivity and independence. Campaigns to hire persons with disabilities have stressed that they can be as productive as those without disabilities. Individuals who cannot produce for some reason are scorned and isolated, cast out, and seen as a burden to the social order. Despite illusions of a safety net, in our highly competitive society people are judged by what they do—not in terms of the resources needed to help them function with some degree of independence.

~

Over the last half century, there has been a noticeable counterforce to this callousness. The compassionate element in U.S. society has shown itself in a number of changes in relation to people who have disabilities, the most significant being the passage of the Americans with Disabilities Act (ADA) in 1990. The changes toward people with disabilities occurred in three phases.

Avoidance and Rejection This early stage viewed those with disabilities as being punished for some sin. Indeed, people were often identified by their disability. Groups in society saw them as deviants in all areas. They were often the butt of jokes. Persons with disabilities were dehumanized and even in some cases sterilized or used as subjects in experiments without their consent. They were offered no services. Families were required to care for them and usually chose to hide them or, if they could not care for them, sent them to institutions. When they did appear outside of the home, they were rejected and avoided. The result of this ostracism on the personal development of the individual with a disability was devastating, with low self-esteem leading to frequent suicidal ideation and many times suicidal behavior.

Tolerance Since the mid-1970s, there has been a recognition of social responsibility for those with disabilities. One effort at greater tolerance is the shift in language: Society is gradually abandoning the term *handicapped people* and more often speaking of "persons with disabilities," thus stressing the person and not the disability. Some groups, notably those with hearing disabilities, have begun to feel empowered and have even spoken of themselves as separate cultures. Curb cuts are becoming more prevalent and have increased access and community participation for wheelchair users. The President's Committee on the Employment of People with Disabilities has brought the issues to the highest level of government. The passage of the ADA was a milestone.

However, major hurdles still remain. Recent data indicate that employment of those with disabilities has not improved significantly despite the ADA ("In 4 years," 1994). Many of those who have disabilities are still living on the margins of the society with resources that are inadequate or barely adequate for survival (many cannot get health insurance, for example). Although access to services has improved, subtle discrimination still remains, even in our helping professions. How often have we heard that persons with mental retardation are not able to profit from psychotherapy, but only need simplistic behavioral management techniques? How frequently have we encountered the belief that persons with physical ailments need only supportive services, not insight? How many times has it been said that engaging the inner life of a person with disabilities is either not possible, not necessary, or not important?

Integration The third, future phase is one of complete mainstreaming and integration. Those with disabilities will not be marginalized, but will be included as an integral part of the social order, able to make decisions about their lives and to obtain the services they need. Services will be based on a careful and thorough evaluation, not on predetermined beliefs. True access to help means availability of *all* services, not just those preselected by individuals with little understanding of persons with disabilities as complex and total individuals. Working with those who have disabilities may be more difficult because it could require contact with families, employers, and other professionals. However, there will be many opportunities for creative interventions to assist the person with disabilities toward leading a useful and satisfying life.

This book is a major step in moving us toward the third phase. It shows how therapists can courageously accept the challenge of working with people who have disabilities. As is evident from the case studies presented, we can learn a great deal about persons with disabilities. Above all, as the authors so vividly show, in our work with those who have disabilities we can learn a great deal about ourselves.

Milton F. Shore, Ph.D., ABPP
Past President
American Orthopsychiatric Association

REFERENCES

Americans with Disabilities Act of 1990 (ADA), PL 101-336. (July 26, 1990). Title 42, U.S.C. 12101 et seq: *U.S. Statutes at Large, 104*, 327–378.
In 4 years, Disabilities Act hasn't improved jobs rate. (1994, October 23). *The New York Times*, p. 1.

Preface

Even, or especially, in the electronic age, books are wonderful things. They invite a kind of immersed, reflective thinking not easily come by in a hectic world. Because of this, they still have some of the magical qualities they had when they were handwritten by monks and scribes. Holding a book is the opposite of watching MTV. Reading a book is like living at a more human pace we are at risk of forgetting.

While thinking about the publication of this book, we were seized by the contradiction between the dynamic acts of thinking and writing that led to its creation and the static quality of words on the written page. We want this book to stimulate thinking and deeper inquiry on the part of its readers, not to be viewed as the final thoughts on the topics it addresses. To work with persons with disabilities requires that the therapist have a deep capacity to bear "not knowing"—to sit with uncertainty, as it were. Perhaps it is this unwillingness to tolerate uncertainty and to bear its attendant anxiety (including anxieties about one's adequacy as a therapist) that leads to so much shoddy therapy and to the dismissal of whole groups of people (in particular, persons with severe mental retardation, autism, and severe and multiple physical disabilities) as unable to benefit from psychotherapy.

To begin this book honestly, and to ground it where it is truly grounded, we need to tell you a bit of our own stories.

Mary Ann Blotzer My current thinking about persons with disabilities has been very much shaped by the disability rights movement and by the rich value base contributed by seminal thinkers such as Burton Blatt, Wolfe Wolfensberger, and Irv Zola. While still in college I had the good fortune to work for Bedford-Somerset (Pennsylvania) Mental Health and Mental Retardation, where I lived with eight women who had recently come home to their community after many years of being confined to institutions. After college and before graduate school, I worked in both residential and day services at a variety of private agencies, including the Arc (formerly the Association for Retarded Citizens).

During these years, I was privileged to have many long dialogues with persons with mental retardation, their families, and the staff who worked with them. I approached these dialogues with the stance described by Bogdan and

Taylor (1982) in their book, *Inside Out*. My goal was to listen unencumbered by theory or structure. Through these conversations and my experience both as service provider and advocate, I became increasingly aware of how incomplete my understanding was. Despite good training, I lacked an adequate conceptual base for thinking about certain issues.

I was also confronted with dilemmas in deciding how to apply certain values as guiding principles. I had seen inexperienced staff use the normalization principle as an excuse for not delivering adequate supports to persons with mental retardation. Even worse, I saw us, in our inexperience and zeal to do the right thing, subordinating individuals to ideologies. I vividly remember one woman who, despite being extraordinarily capable, deteriorated to the point of suicide attempts every time she moved to a more independent setting. She needed relationships with others to function at her best, yet *we* valued "independence" and pushed her into circumstances that were toxic to her. Sometimes, the unintended side effect of our much ballyhooed independence is greater social isolation.

Thankfully, those days of rigid adherence to ideology are falling by the wayside, and I see staff paying greater attention to social and emotional needs. However, there remain obstacles to making services more sensitive to the emotional needs of persons with mental retardation. In Maryland, the state in which I currently work, the state agency that funds and licenses programs for persons with mental retardation requires these agencies to train their direct service staff in certain topics. The required training topics emphasize a mechanistic, reductionistic approach and do not include any focus on the emotional lives of persons with mental retardation. This emphasis reflects the belief in the larger culture that persons with mental retardation lack emotional depth.

I felt my understanding to be incomplete and wanted an expanded conceptual framework for understanding persons with mental retardation. I decided to pursue a graduate degree in a mental health field. After considering the various fields of study, I settled upon social work because it emphasized the person-in-society model. I wanted to comprehend psychological dynamics better, but I also understood the deep role played by social circumstances, especially where persons with mental retardation were concerned.

Some years after my training was completed, I became director of the Developmental Disabilities Program at Community Psychiatric Clinic. My experience there—and the deep, fertile exchanges that I had with my colleagues in the program—formed the backdrop for much of this book.

Richard Ruth When I was a child, there was no polite word for what was the matter with me. Among adults, in fact, there was no word at all—something that I, as a child who sought in words a refuge from the terrifying physical world, found especially disquieting. The adults in my life told me I was smart, wonderful, gifted, and fine. The kids saw it differently.

I was uncoordinated, weak, a "spaz." I didn't stand right or throw right; I couldn't play sports "to save my life" (one of those phrases that captures more than it knows: my life felt damaged, and I was not at all sure I could save it). In a neighborhood of happy children with the simultaneously narrow and unlimited dreams of the well-provided-for, I was not happy and I quickly internalized a sense that my dreams were as unacceptable as I was, and I'd better not pay too much attention to them, for fear of making things worse. Other kids dreamed of more time to ride their bikes; I couldn't ride a bike until I was 12, and I had repetitive dreams of getting rides that would take me the few yards of my awkward and almost intolerably depleting walk from the bus stop to home.

I was not miserable, not without love or gratifications or friends. But I had the lingering sense that my friends didn't like me very much. Part of it was that I was prickly and sharp-tongued and in some ways not all that likeable. Another part was that the things that were wrong with me were not what the social tenor of the times could imagine, or could permit, to be wrong. It was okay not to play a musical instrument; it was *not* okay to "throw like a girl."

And yet, the adults were not lying when they said there was nothing wrong with me. In the words of the time, I had poor motor coordination skills. The words held no transformative potential, and therefore the words made the reality unreal. There wasn't much to do about it—or at least much that made any sense to me.

I was told that, if only I would pay attention and try harder in gym, every thing would work out. It was like asking me to speak a language I didn't speak. I'd try and it wouldn't work. Thankfully, some sane voice at my core told me that I should stop trying before the endless round of failures and frustrations destroyed me. At brief moments, those who loved me knew I was suffering. That was as far as any of us could take it at the time. And, mind you, I had it easy compared to what other people with more visible or severe disabilities have experienced.

Like many children of the 1960s, there came a time when rebellion against what was painful and wounded in my childhood merged with what I raged against in the world. As for my disability, it helped that my coordination improved with puberty and that I discovered one day that my difficulty catching footballs didn't stop me from beating up an obnoxious bully who'd been provoking me for years. Power begets respect. However, as satisfying as it was for the story about the spaz bloodying the nose of the basketball star to wend its way around the neighborhood, I found my real power in becoming politically involved, in finding connections with like-minded people and in the satisfaction of collective action.

I didn't set out to become a therapist. My original desire was to teach school. I wanted to be the kind of social studies teacher that wanders readily from the curriculum, awakens slumbering teenagers to the wonders of the world, and has great conversations with them about the meaning of life. In retrospect, perhaps I was trying to rewrite my childhood history through what I could create with my students. But it didn't work. The high school students I was given to teach, in a poor urban neighborhood, often could not read or write, and the conditions in which they lived had stolen their space for thinking. In the context of their impossible lives, they did not get very worked up about pondering the meaning of life. So I decided that they needed more than a teacher could provide and that I would provide this by becoming a therapist.

Therapy training did not impress me very much at first. It seemed too abstract, too distant from the urban pain that surrounded me and the pain of my own childhood, more dimly remembered through the fog of repression and the social message that "what was wrong with me" did not exist and was best forgotten. But eventually I developed a sense of the possibilities of therapy. Dispossessed memories, like dispossessed people, have loud voices; I found myself developing an allegedly purely intellectual interest in therapeutic work with people with physical disabilities. By the time I discovered what the roots of that were all about, it didn't matter. I was content to live with my calling. And, after living with this calling for a while, it was time to write.

In the ways of the universe, my calling also decided to live with me. As an adult, I've developed diabetes and arthritis, and a car a few years ago decided to un-develop my knees. My disabilities, now several, currently hover on the border of visibility.

~

Giving birth to a book is disconcertingly similar to giving birth to a child. Both processes involve months of mixed excitement and discomfort; odd changes in eating and sleeping habits; coming into closer contact with dreams, longings, and heartfelt beliefs than is usual in day-to-day life; and finally sharing what you hold most intimately with the world.

In both cases, you hope the product of your labor will be a positive addition to the world. We hope you enjoy, and benefit from, this book.

REFERENCE

Bogdan, R., & Taylor, S. (1982). *Inside out: The social meaning of mental retardation.* Toronto: University of Toronto Press.

Acknowledgments

Those of us who do this work understand that conventional notions of independence and dependence mask reality—that in reality we are interdependent and that how effectively we function and how we feel about our lives are deeply affected by the quality of our relationships.

I am fortunate to have been richly sustained in a network that includes family, friends, colleagues, and community—all responding in ways that stretch the boundaries of conventional roles.

Perhaps the best part of this endeavor is the sense of community found with others who are willing to sit with uncertainty and to explore these reaches. My thinking has been stimulated and my spirit nourished by individuals too numerous to mention. I hold them within me and they form the inner landscape from which this book flows.

Many staff persons of residential and vocational programs contributed enormously to my understanding of the dilemmas faced by our patients. Nancie Bauman from the Jewish Foundation for Group Homes, Tammy Denning from CHI–Centers, and Beverly Gordon and Robin Roller from The Arc of Montgomery County deserve special mention. Joyce Lipman and Thyra Packett are parents of adults with mental retardation. Their open-hearted awareness and keen intelligence helped me to stay closely connected to the subjective experience of persons with mental retardation and of their families. The greatest sharing and learning have come from my patients who allowed me to learn what life is like for them.

The value base and mission of the disability rights movement has nourished and inspired me, and I owe a personal debt to Monroe and Joan Karasik, Fred Baughman, Cristy Marchand, Donna Fluke, Jim Ellis, and other individuals too numerous to mention, whose drive and commitment inspire me when my own spirits are flagging.

My mental health colleagues Don Cassidy, Sheila Gart, Bonnie Hetzel, Sandy Jacobson, Chuck Kaelber, Baiba Kelley, Ann Lipp, Ana McNeil, Martie Mitchell, Adele Natter, Shirley Papilsky, Jean Ratner, Rachel Ritvo, Inta Rutins, Carol Toll, Terry Ullman, Judith Willging, and Tim Zwerdling contributed enormously to my understanding and have provided intellectual stimulation and moral support.

Writing a book requires both energy and support from others. I am indebted to my family for providing me with untold moral and practical support, as well as space for thinking. Lastly, my co-author, Richard Ruth, through his combination of clinical wisdom, wit, and realism, made the enterprise both inspiring and inspired. I am excited to see where our ongoing collaboration and friendship will next take us. —M.A.B.

~

Much of my thinking about clinical issues was shaped by a series of professors, administrators, and colleagues who told me my ideas were wrong-headed and dangerous and that my intention to do psychoanalytic psychotherapy with people with disabilities was at best a little flaky and at worst, in one memorable instance, suggestive of personal psychopathology. I would like to thank these persons for helping me to clarify my own thinking and for deepening my lifelong appreciation for the particular value of battle-tested ideas.

I would also like to thank—more warmly—Emmanuel Berman, Rochelle Levine, Rita Gazarik, Florence Samperi, Leon Hankoff, Bernard Murphy, Carol Smith Donovan, Hana Bruml, Anne Coates-Conaway, Zelda Porte, Milton Shore, and Mindel Shore, all of whom have had shaping impacts on my clinical thinking and work.

My experience as a psychoanalytic patient has been essential to my ability to think and to work. I am deeply grateful to the persons who worked with me in this capacity.

Most of what I know, I learned from my work with my patients. The privilege of entering their communities and their hearts and minds is one I value greatly. This work honors their contribution.

One of my greatest discoveries in the process of working on this book is that writing happens in stolen moments, late at night, when other needs press and exhaustion and insight share moments of proximity. No one makes it through such an experience alone. I want to thank my family; my research colleagues, Sara Grusky and Jose Rodriguez; and my friends in the Washington Area Drumming Group for never failing me. To my co-writer Mary Ann Blotzer, whose warm and quiet faith and good friendship are an ongoing source of wonder, I owe a special debt. The pleasure that went into doing this book with her is boundless.

As was impressed on me from an early age, the full responsibility for any errors in my texts is mine alone. —R.R.

~

Mostly we are indebted to our colleages and unindicted co-conspirators on the Developmental Disabilities Team at Community Psychiatric Clinic in Wheaton, Maryland. Our staff meetings and informal discussions were the crucible in which essential issues were distilled and awareness deepened. Our editors at Paul H. Brookes Publishing Co., Victoria Thulman, Elaine Niefeld, and Lynn Weber, crafted this book into shape. To them is owed a special debt as midwives. —R.R. and M.A.B.

For my grandmother, Esther Hubelbank, and
my father, Robert Ruth (R.R.)

This book is dedicated to the more than 6,000 Marylanders
with developmental disabilities who languish on the
state's waiting list for community services, to the
families who care for them, and to those advocates
and elected officials who are working to build a bridge
across the abyss that threatens to swallow hopes,
dreams, and even lives. (M.A.B.)

Sometimes You Just Want to Feel Like a Human Being

1

Toward Basic Principles

Richard Ruth and Mary Ann Blotzer

Telling stories and listening to stories are simultaneously simple and complex acts. It is not, for example, a major production for a parent to tell a child a bedtime story. Yet clearly there are multiple layers of resonance that are also a part of the experience. Through bedtime stories, parent and child bond, moral and emotional teachings are transmitted, and aspects of personality are established and entrenched.

Stories themselves are complex psychological products. There are dynamic tensions between voice and content, which are sometimes mutually reinforcing but sometimes convey the heart of the story through their dissonance. Choices of wording, the occasional unconscious resonance of a phrase, the communication of cultural contents through stock phrases, the presence or absence (conscious or unconscious) of gendered elements of experience—all embody potential meaning. And yet some stories stay with us all our lives—*change* our lives—while others hold little appeal and cross no gates into awareness. Thus, telling and listening to stories can have the odd characteristic of being either a common or a noble experience, or both.

Some of these phenomena may help explain why science has such an ambivalent and ambiguous relationship to storytelling. Scientists want to know about the human experience but usually do not want to hear it the way people tell it. Much traditional science is about a different level of knowledge, one simultaneously more precise and more superficial. With regard to therapy, we face the paradox that our day-to-day work is one of storytelling, but that our training base is in the domain of science. Of course, in today's climate, traditional and nontraditional notions of science interface. This book has close connections to ethnography, qualitative research in behavioral science, and psychoanalytic and systemic therapy approaches. At the same time, many of the contributors to this book have learned from and participated in more quantitative scientific discourses.

~

We begin with a rather disquieting story to frame our discussion of basic principles underlying empowering psychotherapeutic work with people with disabilities. We tell the story not to overwhelm the reader with discomfort or rage, but as a vehicle to help the reader appreciate some aspects of working with disability that are hard to discuss. These issues come into clear focus when they are inadvertently blurted out.

We were sitting in a restaurant eavesdropping on the vacation dinner conversation (it was inevitable—they were loud) of a group of teachers. One, a special education teacher, was giving a really awful version of the "every child can learn" speech: a shallow rendition that, under a liberal guise, obliterated the real difficulties and limitations many children with disabilities experience. One of her dinner partners kept pressing her: What about the more severely affected children who really cannot meet the standard curriculum objectives?

In the manner of animated dinner talk, more-serious-than-usual themes were interrupted by kids seeking quarters for video games and the pleasant meanderings of adult vacation banter. But the line of conversation persisted until another of the teachers interjected: "Well, those other ones, we just put them in the gas chamber." The table exploded in laughter—perhaps nothing more unsavory than teachers venting pent-up tension at the end of a long school year.

This story comes across as almost intolerably raw and powerful, but it captures some deep, important aspects of how people with disabilities are often viewed. The teachers did not seem to us to be exceptionally bad people; their intentions were benign, not at all genocidal. We have both said similar things ourselves in honest and unguarded moments. In a way, what makes the story so powerful is that it seems so common, something that many people involved in some branch of human services might say in a cathartic moment of uncensored frustration. As broadly as we extend our professional embrace, there are some people whom, by virtue of their disabilities, we think of as lying outside it—too damaged, too distant from our visions, too far from the reach of our interventive tools.

And yet this bounding off of therapeutic possibilities is not an uncharged or inconsequential act. When the anonymous teacher's defenses were breached, the unguarded, previously unconscious feelings that emerged had their chilling poetry because they touched something latent.

~

The case studies in this book reflect and examine a position quite different from either of the teachers' alternately naive and pessimistic views. Rather, the writers in this book tend to view disability as a complex, multidimensional variable. It cannot be adequately captured in the neat terms of straightforwardly changeable behavior or curable symptoms, or as something so dark, overwhelming, and impossible that it must be defined as outside the boundaries of the imagination. We tend to embrace the values of curiosity and possibility.

Both therapists and disability rights advocates tend to assert fiercely the primacy of the individual and to be especially wary of overgeneralizations and psychological "laws" whose shallow and problematic base can make for perceptions becoming realities.

~

Disability makes people uncomfortable in a specific way. It evokes primitive fears. Many people do not like thinking about disability because of an unspoken, perhaps unspeakable, fear that, if they do, they may themselves become disabled or will have to confront the weaker parts of themselves—parts often involved with formidable complexities of vulnerability, oppression, identity, unmet need, dependency, confusion, childhood hurts, and shame.

At this deep, unconscious, but nevertheless very real level, charity, denial, and abuse find their common source. All of these behaviors are forms of escape from the reality of disability experience. And when people—especially therapists and other service providers—ignore the reality of disability experience, we compromise our ability to think. Not thinking is particularly dangerous for therapists, because our job is not simply to understand, but to develop understandings sufficiently deep, accurate, and attuned to transformative potentials so that we can help people change. Without this insight, we may use an approach that fails to help or that even hurts.

This book will not detail the long history of abusive treatments that generations of people with disabilities have suffered at the hands of their healers. But it is safe to say that the history is well known, and that its effects are still alive.

Psychotherapeutic work to empower people with disabilities is in its toddlerhood, a stage of hypothesis-generating and small-scale clinical experimentation. The goal at this point is to record and share early experiences in our work and to encourage more widespread reflection and dialogue. Codification and guidelines have yet to be explored. Any attempt to define a basis of principles is treacherous and runs the risks of being premature and inadvertently disrespectful of diverse views and experiences. In this book, we have placed a priority on including diverse voices. This being said, it is often helpful to identify some common principles in an effort to provide cohesion and structure to the reading and thinking experience.

Here is what stands out to us:

1. *People with disabilities have complex inner lives, and a useful way of working can evolve from the struggle to understand their experience.* The notion of an inner life exists in some tension with the general and therapeutic cultures. In the broader culture, it tends to get rejected as an old-fashioned inconvenience and to get briefly embraced on its way to dissolving into narcissism.

Many approaches to therapy treat the question of an inner life similarly. Some behavioral, cognitive, humanistic, and strategic/systemic therapists view inner life as an unscientific illusion, or as a "black box" that has little relevance or meaning for the therapeutic task. Branches of psychodynamic and psychoanalytic thinking closer to contemporary Freudianism tend to focus more on drives and the unconscious than on inner life as a more coherent and holistic phenomenon, or as a useful level of analysis.

Perhaps because disability experience is so inherently violative of social, cultural, and therapeutic preconceptions, many people with disabilities tend to cling rather tenaciously to the importance and prominence of our inner lives. "But that's not how it is for me!" is a common, indignant refrain. Those parts of us that are not allowed much space for living in the world cherish the space for life inside ourselves. And we want to be understood in the particularities, affective contexts, and full range of potentials of who we are.

These ideas about good therapy are specific to work with people with disabilities when the therapist consciously and explicitly retains a value of staying more grounded in a patient/client's inner subjective experience as it relates to disability. We may be particularly attuned to the fact that we do not know very basic things about how an experience of disability plays out in the inner landscape—or that *neither* patient/client nor therapist knows. Whether help or hindrance, the shared assumptions and resultant common routines in work with someone without disabilities are not present. Several writers in this book explicitly reject any move away from this uncertainty at the subjective core. Instead, they value the uncertainty for its potential to generate fertile space for therapeutic work.

~

2. *Social constructionist and disability rights perspectives are viewed as part of the reality of disability experience.* Social constructionism holds that a disability, on a psychological level, exists not (or not solely) within the boundaries of an individual's skin or mind, but is generated in the encounter between an individual and a social ecology. The classic example is that a wheelchair user does not have a functional mobility impairment unless a building lacks a ramp.

The disability rights movement has defined people with disabilities as a *political* minority, many of whose needs should be framed as denied civil rights rather than as unmet goals on a treatment plan. This perspective, which often has met the overt and covert resistance of professional service providers, has won wide support among people with disabilities and is reflected, among other things, in the provisions of the Americans with Disabilities Act, which are visionary (i.e., more a question of vision than of reality) in the rights they grant.

The writers in this book, many of us products of the ranks of the disability rights movement and ourselves persons with disabilities, integrate these concepts in our thinking as clinicians. We are quite familiar with the phenomena of using complaints about the world being unfair as a defense against looking at one's own maladaptive contributions and of the pervasive use of denial of limitations and withdrawal to fantasy as defenses against painful realities that must be confronted. Yet we tend to juxtapose these findings with inquiry about social realities and to create space for both modes and lines of thinking—psychological and social—to coexist in the therapeutic dialogue. Exploring the constellation of fantasies, affects, beliefs, adaptive efforts, and blockages that concern a *real* denial of rights is a subtly but fundamentally different way of thinking about how people with disabilities may think and behave unproductively.

~

3. *Traditional formulations about the psychological impact of disability are inaccurate and should be rejected.* Psychoanalytic thinking has traditionally held that a disability is a kind of psychological loss and that the task confronting a person with a disability is to learn to accept unflinchingly that a loss has occurred—to mourn what has been lost and thus to come to an acceptance of the disability (Fajardo, 1987; Solnit & Spark, 1976).

There are several problems with this way of thinking. Disability implies a loss not just at the moment of acquiring a disability, but repeated insults and "losses" at every turn, when an unaccommodating society causes renewed obstacles and suffering. Disability is a long-term process of working and reworking, not a shift that happens once and for all.

Further, to the extent that society oppresses people with disabilities, it is appropriate to demand rights, not to accept degrading and disempowering restrictions. The deep, subjective experience of disability changes when society acquires collective awareness of disability issues, removes barriers, and establishes reasonable accommodations and when an individual fights to make this happen. Character shapes politics, but politics shapes character, too.

In relational life, people with disabilities must confront not only their own self-limiting patterns, as traditional views counsel, but the extent to which persons without disabilities treat people with disabilities as unwilling containers of their own fears, limitations, and prejudices. In the same way that people of color, members of ethnic groups and immigrants from collectivist cultures, and homosexuals are experienced as threatening because they are experienced as embodying underlying split-off fantasies and impulses, people with disabilities trigger powerful unconscious reactions in persons without disabilities. These reactions are then expressed in behaviors that must be confronted.

It is also important to draw clearer boundaries between phenomena of the inner life and external realities. An unconscious experience of a sensory or motor disability as a loss is qualitatively different from seeing a disability as an objective loss. Wheelchair users may not yearn above anything to be able to walk or be willing to make extensive sacrifices of time, effort, money, and comfort to achieve walking. Those deaf people and blind people who see themselves as different more than disabled may not be expressing denial.

4. *People with different disabilities have more common traits than differences.* The disability rights movement, from the beginning, has emphasized a cross-disability perspective. In part, this is a reaction against the medical/rehabilitation establishment's tendency to reduce personhood to symptom lists, but it is not merely a reactive vision. Neither is it solely a political vision, although a cross-disability perspective has wide appeal from an advocacy point of view.

The more one considers the *psychological* aspects of disability, the more difficult it is to draw clear lines, or any lines, between discrete categories of disability experience. This reality becomes even more compelling when the psychology of disability is considered in a social context, as *no* disability is easily or willingly accommodated in contemporary society. While different people's experiences vary, core dimensions of disability experience—feeling excluded, victimized, different, isolated, unique, "special," or misunderstood, for example—have little to do with the specificity of medical diagnosis or even of functional deficits.

This is not to say that there is no social hierarchy of disability. Powerful collective values tend to judge physical disability as less daunting than cognitive or psychiatric disability, deficits in perception as less incapacitating and stigmatizing than deficits in expressive communication, invisible disability as more benign than visible disability, mild disability as better than severe disability. These are overgeneralizations, and as such are inaccurate, but they serve to communicate a point: that all of these conditions are seen as negative. Thus, while a blind attorney would tend to be perceived on a higher level in the social hierarchy than someone with multiple disabilities working in a sheltered workshop, would anyone really be surprised to hear the opinion that both might envy someone with modest prospects in life but no disabilities?

Again, however, a cross-disability perspective goes beyond a vision of unity among the oppressed. There is at least an emerging sense in disability thinking that a cross-disability view also opens a path toward thinking about common solutions, such as demanding reasonable accommodation as a right, or toward disengaging identity from disability (thus, "people with disabilities" rather than "the handicapped"). As therapists, allowing these possibilities in our own thinking seems to increase the space for creativity in our patients/clients.

~

5. *It is important to counter the pervasive pathologizing of people with disabilities by focusing on strengths and by considering that extreme or unusual personal solutions can be reasonable and adaptive.* Even though there is currently a professional climate where facile rhetoric about human potential is replacing earlier ways of talking about "being limited," there is a gap between what human service providers write about people with disabilities (for example, "there's no telling how far people with mental retardation can go"—a statement with interesting conflicting levels of meaning, i.e., no one should really tell about it) and what is said in case conferences. There, gallows humor is rarely challenged and therapists say what they really think: "This guy will never be a brain surgeon," or, "She should date someone more realistic." The

writers in this book tend to focus more on what such statements deny than on their elements of distorted truth.

We are more likely to view being obstinate as a strength or to validate whining as a survival strategy. We have often been impressed with patients whose stubborn refusal to accept their "objective limitations" has kept them sane or whose lack of cooperation with recommended medical and psychological treatments has been literally lifesaving.

Paul Feuerstein, a therapist who directs an agency that provides mental health services to people with disabilities in New York City, captured the imagination of several of the writers in this book with his concept of "reverent agnosticism" (personal communication, April 1988), meaning that therapists do well to keep open hearts as well as open minds about the "unrealistic" dreams of our patients, that we need to think carefully and hard about what the fantasies of people with disabilities mean before dismissing or obliterating them in therapy. Family therapists have made an important contribution, in most cases inadvertently, to disability thinking by talking about the adaptive function of symptoms when they are viewed in the proper larger context. Thus, as therapists, several of us have often found ourselves supporting life choices of patients/clients that favor comfort over "independence," personal space over full-time repetitive work, and nontraditional options for the intrinsic value of the quest.

6. *Developmentally archaic and mature phenomena coexist in the personalities and behavioral repertoires of people with disabilities; in this sense, disability experience is not a linear phenomenon.* Many schools of contemporary clinical thinking have grown away from notions of psychological growth proceeding through a predictable sequence of stages, and from mechanical notions of cause and effect, in favor of notions of psychological life as less predictable and more complex. Several of us writing in this book have sought to apply these ways of thinking to disability experience.

Thus, we are often more inclined to think about people oscillating between moments when they are stuck and moving forward than older notions of regression and fixation, which have a quality of fixedness that does not seem to fit. Too many of our patients/clients have described experiences that combine success in one area of their life, such as vocational achievement, with devastation in others, such as relationships. Or they describe a pattern of good days and bad days that does not seem shallow or a facet of pathology but is a more essential part of the fabric of their lives.

This is not to say that the writers in this book reject developmental thinking; far from this, it affects us deeply. But it might be fair to say that we tend to see developmental phenomena as much more complex than we were taught to believe. Specifically, we are very skeptical about anything that smacks of developmental inevitability. We have often seen achievements that could not be predicted by the most common developmental equations, and we often *fail* to see people with disabilities achieving some goals, such as family acceptance or predictions of autonomy, which traditional developmental theory predicts. As therapists, we value being open to both sets of these possibilities and to search for countertransferences[1] when they seem unavailable to us.

7. *Empowering therapists work by creating space for thinking and experimenting about disability experience, not by defining disability experience as irrelevant.* Patients/clients with disabilities, when they do find their ways to therapists' offices, are often criticized for dwelling to excess on their disabilities (and at other times for refusing to dwell on them, although that is a separate point). While disability does not shape the totality of the experience of people with disabilities, neither can it be dismissed as a key determinant; and, because there is so little social space or permission for thinking about disability, and there are so many strong presses to think about disability in rigid and narrow ways, so many beliefs about the inherent inevitabilities of disability, it is especially important to create and validate space for thinking about disability, and dialogue about this thinking in therapy.

Effective therapy in this context requires that we carefully distinguish the elements of experience that are within the control and responsibility of an individual from those that flow from society. Interestingly, this parallels a similar development in the thinking of therapists who work with trauma, such as Lenore Terr (1990), who emphasize that assisting patients/clients in identifying what is external may be an essential part of helping them bring the dynamics of their inner lives into clear focus.

In short, the writers of this book maintain that it is important for disability to find its voice; that therapy can be an important place where this can happen; and that messages to the contrary should be viewed with great suspicion.

---

[1]*Countertransference* refers to unconscious reactions in a therapist evoked by unconscious feelings in a patient that the therapist cannot understand clearly.

~

8. *It is vital that therapists be creative and flexible when working with people with disabilities and that at times we resist pressures to be too goal-oriented.* The writers in this book have a variety of theoretical orientations. Cognitive-behavioral, systems, and various schools of psychodynamic/psychoanalytic thinking are represented, and both short-term and long-term treatments are described. Yet many of us find ourselves violating some of the rules we were taught. Not surprisingly, for example, most of us were told in our training that the people we work with are untreatable in psychotherapy. At times this has made our work and our thinking more difficult because we have had to sort out what we embrace and what we reject of our clinical heritage. Nevertheless, we enjoy this creative aspect of our work.

Like all who explore uncharted terrain, we have had to acquire a degree of comfort with being lost—to view this as an inevitable part of the process, rich with possibilities if we can face them and work them through. Thus, we tend to talk about our gaps in understanding, failings, confusions, and limitations somewhat more freely than is common in most clinical texts. Knowing what we do not know seems to play an important function in fostering empathy and may model something vital for our patients/clients as well.

As a corollary to this, we believe that stretches in therapy, sometimes long stretches (in sessions or between sessions), have more an objective of struggling to capture or articulate a feeling, an experience, or idea, rather than simply achieving a straightforward behavioral goal, or correcting a distorted attribution or belief. The uniqueness of the disability experience, contrasted with collective assumptions of our culture, may require extra work and patience to bring certain issues into clear focus.

This is not to say that the therapies described here are unproductive. Rather, several of us have felt the need to deemphasize a goal-oriented approach (hard to avoid in an era of managed mental health care) in favor of an older notion of having a goal of discovering the goals—allowing them to blossom individually. This has often entailed requesting great measures of patience from our patients/clients, their families and support workers, funding sources, and ourselves.

~

9. *Therapists of people with disabilities may need to accept more responsibility than is traditional for realities outside the consulting room and at times may legitimately adopt directive stances, become concerned with practical matters, and engage in advocacy efforts.* While this may be an area

where there is less agreement among the authors, we probably all agree that we think about outside-the-office issues more than therapists who work with other populations. It would be impossible, for example, to go into therapy with a person with a disability without educating ourselves about the physical nature of the disability. (At the same time, it would also be necessary to put these notions aside in favor of listening carefully for idiosyncrasies of an individual's own subjective and historical experience.)

Many of us also go several steps beyond this. All the writers in this book who discuss work with people with developmental disabilities, for example, have contact with different categories of caregivers. Some describe becoming involved in the arrangement of concrete services, in advocacy efforts (sometimes impassioned and protracted), and in therapeutic styles that combine psychoeducation with more exploratory work. We find little difficulty in doing this (or, perhaps more modestly, less difficulty than we or others may have predicted).

Part of this work flows from very practical concerns—people with no money, food, or place to live, and *particularly* people with disabilities in these situations, will have little availability for therapy. But the concerns are not solely practical. Entering into an advocacy role for patients and helping them secure basic services can re-create a core dynamic of how the patient/client interacts in the outside world, a variant of the classical transference experience, and therapists find this an exceptionally valuable source of leverage for the more central therapeutic tasks of reconstructing and understanding what goes wrong in repetitive patterns.

10. *Issues of self-determination and locus of control need to be explicitly addressed.* People with disabilities are often, not wholly incorrectly, described as tending to be more guarded, suspicious, sensitive to slights, and zealous about protecting their right to decide than persons without disabilities. While clinical thinking in general has evolved toward less paternalistic and more democratic stances, there is often reluctance to extend these ways of thinking to people with disabilities. Challenging unrealistic beliefs and behavior patterns seen as counterproductive is often emphasized, subtly or not so subtly.

What is stressed in several of the cases in this book is the value of asking, as an integral and sometimes central aspect of the therapy, questions about who controls what. The value lies in the dialogue, in making the issue dynamic, rather than focusing on one or the other assumption (i.e., that the therapist sets the rules and embodies the wisdom or that the patient/client does and that parallel phenomena go on with other persons in positions of power in the lives of our patients/clients).

At other points, however, clear emphasis is placed on meticulous and fundamental respect for the right of the patient/client to have full control over life choices and decisions. In part this approach is offered as a counterweight to traditional social assumptions that move in opposite directions. In part it relates to a radical view, embedded in much traditional clinical thinking but often honored in the breach, that therapy has its greatest impact when the patient/client is brought into the fullest measure of agency. This takes on a unique slant in work with people with disabilities, who often have internalized messages that they are even less entitled than most to pride of place in their life decisions.

Decisions about when in therapy issues of self-determination need to be questioned and when they need to be placed beyond question remain quite challenging. Perhaps, as Winnicott (1980) has suggested is often the case, this is one of the inherent paradoxes of therapeutic work: that both mutually exclusive assumptions are in some way simultaneously true.

~

11. *Disability is not just an obstacle to be eliminated. It has a political, social, and evolutionary role that is positive; it can be celebrated and enjoyed. Part of the value of treatment is in bringing out this aspect of disability experience.* Often more implied than stated in the case studies in this book is the sense that sometimes disability has a value, and a positively invested value, contrary to social assumptions that it is a burden to be obliterated, destroyed, and forgotten. This is *not* to say that the authors here buy into the more facile views that disability is in some sense a "gift"; the clarity with which the deep pain of disability achieves a voice here is unmistakable.

Rather, the sense is that disability is not necessarily a mistake of the universe and that disability experience takes its shape not because of simple ignorance or prejudice, which can be easily rooted out by education and good will, but because of much deeper phenomena. Many writers here endorse the view that society creates disability not randomly or accidentally, but with some element of logic or intent. The way people with disabilities are viewed and treated may serve as a check against the aspirations of other disempowered social strata, bolster patriarchal family structures, or serve as a press toward social conformity. These larger social currents may in turn become internalized in people with disabilities, making for character defenses and self-limiting beliefs that can be usefully examined in therapy. For example, many people with disabilities internalize desires to "act normal" that are in conflict with their deepest wishes, so as not to incur further social opprobrium. Furthermore, in ways that may roughly parallel the unimaginable achievements that some patients/clients in this book obtain, quite possibly societies can learn where their limitations lie and think about how they may be overcome, in part through their interactions with people with disabilities.

Perhaps the farthest shore of this line of thinking is approached when we read in some of these case studies about people who embrace their disabilities with fierce pride and unmistakable pleasure. Can it be that, precisely through understanding and embracing disabilities, people can *in some circumstances* find elements of human potential that would otherwise have gone undiscovered or undeveloped? If so, what are these circumstances? What is being talked about here is not success *in spite of* disability, but disability *as* a kind of success. The clearest example is in the liberating potential of Deaf culture, described by Don Cassidy's client, but there are other examples as well. This point is subtle and easily shades into beliefs the writers in this volume definitely would not share. But perhaps, as one of the less clear elements of our collective thinking, it is among those most rich with potential, and available for further exploration and development.

This is as far as we feel safe in going with common principles. While several of the writers in this book converge in their thinking in other areas, we would not want to overemphasize the convergences. Perhaps the most important wellspring of creativity lies in the differences. Besides, the writers represented here are walking advertisements for empowerment and assertiveness; all speak their piece without much reservation.

We should acknowledge, however, that this book has been percolating for many years. It arises in large part from discussions in the Study Group on Disability of the American Orthopsychiatric Association (ORTHO), in which several of the writers in this book have participated. ORTHO is an interdisciplinary organization of mental health and allied professionals in the United States and Canada. It is deservedly renowned as a hospitable medium for innovative thinking in many areas of clinical practice and social policy. ORTHO formed a Study Group on Disability in 1986, which has presented annual programs on empowering psychotherapy with people with disabilities and related topics since that time. Several of us—both coauthors of this chapter, Don Cassidy, Adele Natter, and Jean Ratner—have also had the pleasure of working together for the past several years in the Developmental Disabilities Program of Community Psychiatric Clinic, a nonprofit agency in the suburbs of Washington, D.C.

As is often the case with such long-fermenting discussions, we have found it necessary to focus more on releasing this book than on ensuring its completeness. There is more to be said, for example, about the history of some of the work and ideas discussed here. We are too much in the middle of the work to have a clear perspective on its precedents; that can come later. For now, we are eager for you to read our stories.

REFERENCES

Americans with Disabilities Act of 1990 (ADA), PL 101-336. (July 26, 1990). Title 42, U.S.C. 12101 et seq: *U.S. Statutes at Large, 104*, 327–378.

Fajardo, B. (1987). Parenting a damaged child: Mourning, regression, and disappointment. *Psychoanalytic Review, 77*, 19–43.

Solnit, A., & Spark, M. (1976). Mourning and the birth of a defective child. *Psychoanalytic Study of the Child, 17*, 523–537.

Terr, L. (1990). *Too scared to cry: Psychic trauma in childhood.* New York: Harper.

Winnicott, D.W. (1980). *Playing and reality.* London: Penguin.

2

On Sitting with Uncertainty

Treatment Considerations for Persons with Disabilities

Mary Ann Blotzer and Richard Ruth

This book attempts to illustrate the complexities of psychotherapy among individuals with disabilities. Using case studies, we strive to identify, name, and examine these issues. What is remarkable, as one reads these case studies, is the extent to which all the writers struggle with multiple realities. While working with and thinking about their patients, they try to keep many factors in mind—internal subjective reality and its intersection with social reality; considerations about the patient's health status and its implications; a sense of which neuropsychological capacities seem relatively intact and those that seem compromised, and whether such compromise is organic or perhaps mediated by psychodynamic factors; as well as the quality of the individual's relationships with kin, friends, and service providers. These factors, among others, form both the matrix in which the patient lives and the matrix that must be considered during the conduct of therapy.

Although we tackle specific issues, there will always be uncertainties. Ideally, we should strike the delicate balance of labeling some problems and allowing for ambiguity in therapy regarding others. At the same time, acknowledging and exploring the dynamic tensions that accompany these issues can unleash tremendous energy. When the real factors at work are recognized and explored in their full complexity, the transformative potential of therapy can be realized. From a deep awareness of this position, we invite the reader to consider the following dynamic tensions in the treatment of persons with severe disabilities.

~

Intellectual "capacity" can vary as a function of anxiety, conflict, trauma, defense, or other variables. The case of Wendy (Chapter 5) illustrates this phenomenon especially powerfully. Soon after Wendy's mother died, the psychiatrist who saw her monthly for medication management referred her to a therapist who visited her at home. After a few visits, that therapist phoned the psychiatrist with the pronouncement that Wendy was "unable to benefit from therapy" because she was unable to talk about her feelings. Her psychiatrist then referred her to the author. Although the story of Wendy's therapy illustrates how mistaken this pronouncement was, it also illustrates how ponderous the first year of her therapy was. Nearly all Wendy would say during those first months was, "My mother died. My father's in a nursing home." She never amplified on these statements nor did she acknowledge any feelings surrounding these facts. For the first year of her therapy, Wendy spoke in such a concrete and rigidly repetitive fashion, and was so constricted in what she did say, that her therapist thought she was much more organically impaired and limited than she really was. During that first year, Wendy's massive anxiety and rigid defensive structure consistently inhibited both her intellectual functioning and emotional availability. As a result, she had few resources to bring to therapy. She could neither talk about her feelings nor attempt to solve problems. The therapy felt tedious and lifeless because Wendy's self was in hiding. Her rigidity and repetitiveness squeezed all the life out of the room. But this was the only way she could cope with massive losses without decompensating into psychosis. Over time, as her rigidity eased, she showed greater flexibility, greater emotional availability, and even greater intelligence than one would have earlier thought possible.

Wendy's case also illustrates what appears to be a reciprocal relationship between intellectual capacity and defensive strategies. Not only does her limited capacity mitigate against the development of more sophisticated, flexible defenses, but when under stress these defenses intensify, leaving her with less of her intellectual faculties available for function.

Just as stress affects intellectual functioning, so does it affect ego functioning, including reality testing. Certain ego functions (such as the ability to distinguish reality from fantasy, anticipation and planning, and defense mechanisms) may be less firmly established and may desert the patient under stress. On more than a few occasions, we have seen persons with mental retardation demonstrate psychotic symptoms that reflected the patient's profound disorganization when overwhelmed and did not indicate a biologically based psychotic disorder. In this sense we view ego functioning not as a mechanical interaction among structures, but as something more authentically psychological and dynamic and less rigidly separated from instincts, drives, fantasies, and social forces than some theorists would hold.

Finally, Valerie Sinason and her colleagues at the Tavistock Clinic at London have discussed the phenomenon of "secondary mental handicap," whereby individuals with mental retardation consciously or unconsciously intensify their mental handicap. The mechanism serves a variety of functions, from providing a source of control over the uncontrollable (having a mental handicap) to encapsulating anger (Sinason, 1986).

~

Distinguishing the capacities that seem compromised from those that seem intact and acting accordingly can enhance both empathy with the patient and the quality of treatment. This approach is perhaps a variant of the deficit model. But it rejects the absolutism of both the deficit model as well as of the developmental model with its optimistic emphasis on steady growth through maturation and experience. The deficit model was and remains a key underpinning of approaches that segregate persons with disabilities and denies them their full civil and human rights. It often leads to the restriction of opportunities for growth. A vicious cycle soon results with the person's presumed "deficits" taken as justification for restricting his or her opportunities and the denial of opportunities, leading to further deficits.

In response to this and to the movements of segregation and institutionalization created by the deficit model, the developmental model has become more widely accepted. But when we deny the seriousness and permanence of the disabilities that we see, as well as the feelings they evoke in us, the developmental model can fail. We risk making unrealistic expectations for change on the part of persons with disabilities and failing to empathically acknowledge just how limiting and immutable certain aspects of an individual's disability can be.

The deficit model can be especially useful in helping caregivers—whether rehabilitation professionals, job coaches, residential staff, or parents—determine which abilities, personality traits or tendencies, and limitations are relatively immutable as opposed to those that are likely to change with rehabilitation, good caregiving, therapy, and self-control. Freeing patients from the unrealistic expectations of their caregivers can have powerful therapeutic benefits for both the patient and the caregiver.

Sometimes the "fixed" part relates to personality organizations. An example was Henry, a man with mild mental retardation and a narcissistic personality disorder, who lived in a group home and was seen with his house counselor by one of the authors. The house counselor was terribly frustrated and chronically disappointed in Henry because he "always had to be the center of attention" and was "totally insensitive to the feelings of others"—qualities that are quite consistent with a narcissist. The counselor, a bright young man who really wanted to do right by his clients, needed just a few sessions of consultation to alter his approach to the client. For example, a typical sticking point had always been when another resident of the group house was the center of attention, perhaps because it was his birthday or because he was sick. In the past, the house counselor would expect Henry to show appropriate empathy and would become frustrated by Henry's "insensitivity" when he did not. Once he understood the narcissistic character structure, he began to respond differently to Henry.

At times he would prepare Henry in advance whenever another resident would be the center of attention, taking Henry aside to sympathetically acknowledge, "I know it'll be hard on you to see Martin getting all those presents." This altered approach led to a much improved relationship between Henry and his house counselor and also to improvements to Henry's well-being. This came about because the house counselor shifted from viewing Henry's lack of empathy and self-centeredness as character flaws that could be remedied by self-control to viewing these qualities as part of an ingrained pattern of personality organization that would require significant treatment to alter.

Another pertinent example was the case of a man our team had treated who had a history of head injury and an unspecified psychotic disorder. He was referred for "disruptive behavior"—a catch-all phrase. When seen for his initial appointment, he was certainly disruptive—shouting in the waiting room, crying, pacing, and barely able to participate in the interview. The supervisor of his assisted living program explained that the man was this agitated because he had run out of tobacco 2 days prior and did not have the money to buy more. Upon interviewing both the supervisor and the man himself, it became apparent that the major contributing factor to the man's disruptive behavior was that for months now, he had been cycling between nicotine intoxication and nicotine withdrawal. Largely because of deficits associated with his head injury, he was unable to pace his nicotine intake so that he would not run out until he had the money to buy more. Because he had deficits in his ability to plan ahead and to control his intake, and because the staff did not want to violate his rights by controlling his access to tobacco, the man was suffering terribly. He was unable to concentrate or to maintain a stable mood. Our intervention in this case mainly consisted of documenting the man's deficit through neuropsychological testing and meeting with the patient, his staff, and personnel from the human rights monitoring agency to discuss a plan for providing him with the support he needed to manage his nicotine intake to avoid the extremes of intoxication or withdrawal. Had we not talked with this man and his staff about his deficits in the areas of planning ahead and regulating his nicotine—deficits that were due to his head injury—we would have ill-served him. Although this is a dramatic example, it illustrates the importance of recognizing deficits and planning appropriately.

Similarly, therapists can find it helpful to isolate those "capacities" that seem more flexible and apt to develop from those that seem more rigid and deficient. Sometimes these will be as clear-cut as in the example just given. Other times these faculties will be more subtle, and we will be less sure of their underlying cause or chronicity. Nonetheless, this way of assessing a patient's capabilities is an important aid to adequately understanding and planning for the patient, while communicating empathy to the patient. Our patients need us to understand what feels most difficult for or intractable to them. This does not mean that we never expect change in the more rigid or deficient capacities, but that we approach these limitations respectfully.

An example of this approach might be R.J. (Chapter 6), who has a leg injury felt to be irreparable and walks with a limp, pain, and limited endurance, but who still walks and often minimizes his abilities, externalizes responsibility for his problems, and gives up far too easily. For a long time, friends and rehabilitation professionals told him he could walk more if he would only try—that he should give up his cane and his attitude, as it were. It took a lot of work in therapy before R.J. could work through his complex of fantasies and resistances enough to see a rehabilitation doctor for an objective opinion. The opinion was that the prognosis was negative and that R.J. would do best to limit his walking and use a wheelchair for activities requiring distance and endurance. Yet another long stretch of therapy was needed to help R.J. accept this pronouncement.

An important note of caution: Talking about deficits in this way is not a value-neutral enterprise. Talking about deficits evokes a host of reactions, including tendencies to restrict, to become punitive, and to protect in ways that demean and isolate. An individual's supposed "deficits" can also become a self-fulfilling prophecy when treatment teams restrict the opportunities available to the individual, in the interests of "protecting" him from his deficits. We perhaps have an obligation to concurrently discuss the supports and opportunities that will enable the person to function successfully in the real world. Without such a concurrent discussion to plan supports, the discussion of deficits may be used to further isolate and restrict the person.

~

The reciprocal relationship between mental health and social supports may be even stronger where persons with severe disabilities are concerned. Fundamentally, the Americans with Disabilities Act of 1990 (PL 101-336) is about the right of inclusion and the right to reasonable accommodations to ensure inclusion. Without such rights, persons with severe disabilities are relegated to a twilight zone, unable to fully assume adult roles and receive the gratification and opportunities that such roles bring. One needs little imagination to consider that an individual's mental health is adversely affected by not being able to work, by not having accessible transportation, or by being denied participation in most aspects of community life by architectural and other barriers.

Some individuals with severe disabilities require more than reasonable accommodations and the elimination of barriers. They require ongoing services, yet may face governments unwilling to adequately fund these services. The authors work in Maryland, a state with one of the longest waiting lists for community support services for persons with mental retardation and one that ranks in the bottom 10 of the 50 states for spending on developmental disability services as a percentage of per capita income. Consequently, we frequently see young adults with no prior history of mental disorder presenting with major depression, depression with psychotic features, elective mutism, and other serious disorders that are directly attributable to Maryland's inability to adequately provide adult services.

Once their educational entitlement ends in their 21st year, these young adults have no guarantee that they will have a place to go during the day, work that gives them a sense of accomplishment and identity, and a home away from their parents. To both them and their parents, the future looms as a black hole that threatens to swallow their hopes and dreams, and even their sense of self. Depressive disorders are common.

The sense of hopelessness and helplessness that many families feel is both objectively and subjectively real. Faced with limited funds, Maryland's policy has been to prioritize funding for adults with developmental disabilities—first priority goes to those who are homeless or about to become homeless due to the death of their parents. Practically, this means that parents in their 50s, 60s, 70s, and even 80s are still caring for their now-adult children. Such situations can run counter to the developmental impetus of individuals and to family life and social norms.

Children seek greater autonomy from their parents as they age, and parents look to eased demands as their children age. Because the reality for caregiving families runs counter to these needs, development is often stymied. Emotional disorders commonly result. Therapy in these circumstances involves an approach that acknowledges the very real truth that both the family's and the individual's distress are substantially caused by failures of the social "safety net." There are many layers to the feelings associated with this acknowledgment. For many families, the failure of government to adequately provide for persons with developmental disabilities confirms the notion that persons with disabilities are a devalued group. The emotional turmoil surrounding these issues is complex and requires a therapist who is willing to bear its examination without resorting to false reassurances or exhortations to cope more effectively. Therapy is based in large part on diminishing distortion and seeing truth, as difficult as that might be.

Distinctions between dynamic and supportive therapy may be artificial, with the therapist using elements from both during interviews. While psychoanalytic concepts can contribute enormously to our understanding of all persons, including those with disabilities, unreflective applications of classic psychoanalytic techniques may be wholly inappropriate to the treatment of many persons with disabilities. Therapists sometimes forget just how ambiguous the therapy hour can be to persons who are unfamiliar with therapy. This ambiguity can be ego taxing, and the very neutral therapist can be seen as aloof and unsupportive. Sometimes the therapist will need to strengthen vulnerable ego functions by being especially direct and unambiguous. At other times, the therapist will adopt a more dynamically oriented stance to generate greater awareness on the part of the patient and to provide more "space" for treatment designed to foster deeper understanding and change on the patient's part.

Therapists need to consider carefully what their patients need at any moment in the interview. Sometimes probing is needed to deepen the level of inquiry. Sometimes an appropriately timed interpretation is effective. At other times direct information or feedback yield results. Such candor can strengthen vulnerable structures or defenses that would be weakened or left unsupported by a more classically analytic stance. Several of the cases in this book illustrate this oscillation between more dynamically oriented and supportively oriented comments from the therapist, all paced to the needs of the patient at that particular time. In some ways this is nothing new. It is what skillful, helpful therapists have done all along. But it bears particular mention here because the practical realities in the lives of persons with disabilities are more apt to become the province of therapy.

Therapists may need to actively involve themselves in the larger systems that affect their clients' lives. These larger systems may be the deliberate focus of treatment. The lives of persons with severe disabilities are often deeply embedded in social and service systems networks. It is not uncommon for therapists to see persons with severe disabilities who receive services from an assisted housing program, work in supported employment, and maintain active involvement with their families. The quality of these services and of relationships with service providers and family members can significantly affect the client's emotional functioning. These services and relationships, when at their best, can enhance emotional well-being. When at their worst, they can engender psychopathology. To be at their best, service system personnel need to fully understand the client, and the service must be flexible enough to individualize its supports, based upon the needs of the client. Yet sometimes key personnel lack an empathic understanding of the client, or their needs and feelings prevent them from responding appropriately. In addition, service agencies may have rules and procedures that run counter to the client's needs. On these occasions, the therapist may need to step in with interventions designed to effect change in the system or to encourage the staff to respond more appropriately. This is a legitimate province of therapy, but the therapist must recognize how this involvement affects the therapy.

Issues of therapist neutrality, therapeutic alliance, and client confidentiality must be carefully assessed to develop the appropriate stance to best meet the needs of the patient and the exigencies of the situation. How will contact with others affect the therapeutic alliance? If the therapist listens to the assisted housing provider's criticism of the client, will the client then view the therapist as biased against him or her? How will it affect their ability to work together in therapy? Will the client still feel the safety necessary to honestly explore his or her life? Will the therapist have crossed over a line and not be able to maintain a neutral, exploratory stance? There is no one, right answer. The answer depends on the judgment and humanity of the therapist.

Our work with patients has demonstrated the importance of allowing the client's dynamics and the content of the therapy to determine the scope of our involvement in any given case. Some individuals need us to maintain strong boundaries and actively avoid involvement with the other important figures in their lives. As recipients of publicly funded services, their "clienthood" exposes them to constant scrutiny and regular invasions of privacy. Groups of individuals meet regularly to talk about them; they are constantly being assessed and their responses documented. One of us (M.A.B.) vividly remembers working with a woman who spent years in a residential school and who had recently moved to an assisted living program near her parents. Both the woman's parents and program staff had difficulty accepting her need for psychological space and constantly assaulted her with pressure and questions. She desperately needed her therapist to remain as aloof as possible from the other individuals in her system. Furthermore, because she had always been psychologically chased, prodded, and probed, she needed her therapist to be deliberately unintrusive in the conduct of her therapy so that she could have the space to explore her life on her own terms and schedule. Despite intense pressure from her parents and residential staff, the therapist maintained this stance. To have done otherwise would have violated both her rights and the therapist's code of ethics and would have been bad therapy.

But there are individuals who want and need us to communicate with their families and program staffs. Indeed, this communication can advance the goals of the therapy. The cases of Sebastian (Chapter 7), Amy (Chapter 10), and Wendy (Chapter 5) illustrate this need. Far from harming the therapeutic alliance, these individuals felt comforted, relieved, and supported by their therapists' involvement with larger systems.

Be guided by ideology, and beware of ideology. This last paradox is especially fitting. Ideologies based upon a coherent value base have guided most of the significant movements that led to expanded rights and services for persons with disabilities. Regardless of the specific ideologies, each one has empowered a disempowered group and truly holds transformative potential. Thinking differently about an issue actually can lead to the issue being transformed and previously unseen potentials opening up.

Therapists who do the kind of work described in this book must be aware of these ideologies as much as they must be aware of different schools of psychological thinking. Therapy is never a neutral, value-free enterprise. The therapist who views disability simply as a loss to be gotten over will approach therapy very differently from one who appreciates disability in all its contexts—social, political, and intrapsychic.

As therapists who have a foot in both the disability rights movement and in the consulting room, we pay attention to ideology as well as the patient's subjective experiences. But we give primary attention to the person's subjective experience, even when this conflicts with the orthodoxy of the times. For example, one of us (M.A.B.) remembers a woman who had mild mental retardation and lived in a small home staffed by the local assisted-living agency. The woman had many skills and did not need live-in staff assistance. Yet whenever the program moved her to a more independent setting, she deteriorated rapidly and became depressed and suicidal. For this woman, the consequence of greater independence was greater social isolation. Ultimately, the program's staff recognized this need and planned appropriately.

On numerous occasions our patients have reminded us that they are individuals first and may or may not want to "get with the program" by leading a life prescribed by the prevailing ideology. We supported this even when their stories conflicted with the sacrosanct ideologies of the times. To do otherwise would be to subordinate the individual to the ideology.

As you read the case studies that follow, it is helpful to remember some of the challenges we just described concerning psychotherapy with persons who have disabilities. Remarkably, most of the crises discussed in the case studies were resolved despite the obstacles. In all cases, the therapists had to use a unique blend of approaches to fit the demands of each person and situation. Clearly, each of these therapists illustrates the willingness to sit with uncertainty and to pay primary attention to the subjective experience of each patient.

REFERENCES

Americans with Disabilities Act (ADA) of 1990, PL 101-336. (July 26, 1990). Title 42, U.S.C. 12101 et seq: *U.S. Statutes at Large, 104*, 327–378.

Sinason, V.E. (1986). Secondary mental handicap and its relationship to trauma. *Psychoanalytic Psychotherapy*, 2(2), 131–154.

3

Rex

Leaving Therapy Unresolved

Richard Ruth

Shortly after I began my private practice, a team of wise colleagues—a school psychologist, a school placement professional, and a youth services worker—conspired to refer to me an 8-year old South American immigrant boy with visual disabilities. They believed that the child, Rex, needed more intensive psychotherapy than the public system had been able to provide him. The family received welfare, so they could not pay my fees. The referral was made in the finest tradition of professionals begging sympathetic colleagues to do difficult work for free, something I suspect everyone with an honest heart who has worked with people with disabilities has done occasionally.

Rex and I worked together for almost 5 years, twice a week. The therapy was conducted in Spanish, in which we both have native fluency. My desire to write about our work stems from a wish to convey the reality of a Hispanic boy with a disability—not to make him a stereotype or deny his individuality, but with a sense that his story has wider implications. My other reason for telling Rex's story is more personal—a desire, perhaps a need, to share the thinking behind my attempt to work with him therapeutically; an attempt that, in retrospect, did not accomplish what I had hoped it might.

~

Rex often came into the office exhausted. The intense emotional demands of his school day, the intensity of his feelings about being in therapy, and the partially hidden thoughts and feelings therapy evoked for him would physically and emotionally drain his energy. He even had trouble sitting upright during therapy. I also had the impression that he felt he could let go in his therapy sessions, where he knew he was safe and respected and had my attention completely focused on him. Further—as if this all were not complicated enough—Rex did not experience home as very nurturing. He was angry at his mother, a chronically overwhelmed woman whom he loved and respected but experienced as maddeningly self-absorbed. He was often angry and aggressive toward his siblings, both younger. In their aspects of helplessness and neediness, they seemed to remind him, intolerably, of his own deficits. Thus, part of the sleepiness that overcame Rex the moment he came into the office was probably related to his awareness that all too soon he would have to go home.

Although there were several inviting places in the office where he could stretch out, Rex allowed himself few comforts. He usually sat on a stool near my feet, hunched over. Despite his problems, Rex was meticulous about his appearance. Rex was handsome, with a facial expression part sultry, part vacant, and a trendy haircut with lots of mousse to create a sense of artistic disarray. He often wore stonewashed jeans, knockoffs of middle-school high fashion, brand-name sneakers well exceeding the family budget, and a Ninja Turtle T-shirt.

Rex's favorite toy, among the many available, was a ratty blue Nerf ball, hand-sized. He had three ball games that he liked. In "volleyball," we took turns—inevitably, he got more turns than I—trying to smack the ball so that it hit the wall behind the other player. If it did, you got a point. You got to try to block the ball if you could. In "dodge ball," we took turns throwing the ball at each other; if it hit, you got a point. You could either dodge the ball or try to catch it; catching it did not count as a hit. Then there was an unnamed game, where you tried to hit the ball up in the air as many times as you could. Sometimes we took turns playing this game, although Rex preferred playing alone while I watched him, with the never-stated but always-present expectation that I would keep track of how many times he hit the ball.

I think about these games largely in the psychoanalytic terms of projection and introjection. *Projection* refers to people expelling parts of themselves they cannot tolerate and placing them for transformative safekeeping into another person. *Introjection* refers to taking back from another person, such as a therapist, a desired quality. "Taking heart" from a role model would be an example. These phenomena are odd-sounding but not uncommon. They happen regularly in everyday life, and they happen a lot in therapy.

The ball was a kind of neutral medium for Rex, into which he projected a wealth of feeling. Sometimes the unconscious intention seemed to be for me to "hold" the feelings he hurled at me with the ball, so that, after I caught the ball, the feelings became metabolized in me as if I were a kind of emotional dialysis machine, able to detoxify feelings that were too threatening for Rex to tolerate. When I threw the ball back and Rex could catch it, he could take introjected possession of his own material in a more benign and usable form. At other times, Rex seemed to turn in on himself in the ball play, and it became almost intolerably boring for me. Perhaps I felt this way because the unconscious feelings—of terror, woundedness, impotence, and being overwhelmed—that accompanied this regressive retreat were subtly being projected into me. I experienced them as intolerable, empathically, as Rex did. There was always a dual quality to the ball play—resisting talking and explicit awareness, on the one hand; on the other, symbolically depicting Rex's inner world.

~

Some 2 years into the therapy, when he was almost 11, Rex came in and sat on my footstool, probably sensing that I would want to start out talking to him for a while, and perhaps to give the impression that he might even allow for some conversation. On that day, I stayed quiet for a few minutes; my sense was that his body posture subtly relaxed. He seemed less hypervigilant, less tense, and less removed. After a while I asked him some simple questions—how his day went, what was on his mind. His answers were mumbled, brief, and not particularly revealing, but the interpersonal space was ritually marked.

Rex asked, "Can we play?" He had heard a million times that he could do whatever he wants in the therapy sessions; he did not have to ask. Perhaps the question was a form of respect, another ritual marking, or a way of saying that there was an element of intentionality and mindfulness present, making playing in therapy different, special—*therapeutic*.

On that day, Rex began with the hitting-the-ball-in-the-air game. His play was intense; soon he started to breathe heavily, almost reaching the point of asthmatic breathing. He wore his glasses. For years he had resisted this, but lately he was wearing them more often, which implied some degree of acceptance of his disability in a still-obscure fashion.

The quality of Rex's play oscillated between several poles. Sometimes he showed intense mental focus, concentrating remarkably, accommodating visually, and moving with grace. It was as if someone poured water on him and he turned alive. I thought, with mixed emotion, how close he was to puberty—happy that his development was in some ways progressing yet overwhelmed with the deficits he was bringing with him to this developmental turning point. At other times, his play became silly, doing things he knew would not work, as a form of tension-release as well as self-deprecation. This latter trait never stayed hidden too long, because when Rex felt the least bit ineffective, he began to scowl and mutter, his face darkening visibly. The third pole was one of exhaustion. At these times he became listless, unfocused, draggy.

This was a good day. Rex hit the ball 81 times on his best turn, one of his best performances. He smiled broadly when he asked me the number on his better turns; when I answered, he jumped in the air and made proud gestures and macho noises. The effect was one of satisfied self-efficacy and narcissism. From time to time, I offered an interpretive monologue. Rex did not actively resist this, but did not engage with it either. My sense was that he had trouble tolerating an active interpretive stance, but that something was registering in his unconscious, that his filtering out represented the workings of a nascent filter—a positive advance for Rex.

Some 20 minutes into the session, Rex asked me to play volleyball. Most of his hits were powerful and effective, although occasionally he hit a "trick" shot with little chance of winning him a point; I found myself playing hard and well, not giving him a handicap. I noticed that he took some pleasure in my winning. I also sensed that he was pulling this kind of play from me, related to the workings of projective identification. Rex identified with a quality, originally his own, that he had projected into me. Earlier on in the therapy, any time I won a point, Rex would say, "Let's start." He would begin the game all over again, cheating, lying, and becoming frustrated any time I won a point. During this session, however, his frustration tolerance was better; the workings of a desire for mastery were apparent—good things, gains of therapy. At the same time, this almost-teenager was saying very little, hitting a ratty Nerf ball endlessly up and down, back and forth. Upon reflection, I wonder if my frustration showed and how Rex reacted to it.

The volleyball game ended 7 minutes before the end of the session. This created a delicate situation—Would he ask to play something that he knew would take too long and then get angry with me when I kept to the schedule. Would his exhaustion return more intensely, with Rex assuming a turtle posture? Would he talk for a while?

At this particular session, Rex declined to play and sat on the sofa. I asked if he would like to chat for a while, and he said yes; but again, as at the beginning of the session, he did not say very much. We sat, largely in silence; I volunteered a couple of interpretative comments about his play today and then asked some questions. I got very little verbal response and a few stretches of closed eyes. Rex's body posture was relaxed, however; when his eyes were open, his face looked alive, like he was thinking about things and thinking productively. This was a major improvement for this boy who used to be unable to think much about his life or stay in any kind of touch with his feelings, and still sometimes regressed to an unreachable posture. There was never any eye contact, polite greeting, proud erectness, or softened vulnerability. Rex seemed aware of my presence across from him, looking at me from time to time, smiling once or twice, not resisting eye contact. This may have been part of the process of containing, an unconscious process, whereby my presence provided a receptacle for Rex's unconscious material, in a subtle but powerful way. It facilitated the unfolding of his awareness and his tolerance of a higher level of behavioral functioning.

At the end of our time, I informed Rex that our session was completed for the day, and Rex calmly and pleasantly walked toward the door and said goodbye. He always did this twice—once before leaving the office and once between the door to my office and the second door, about a yard away, leading out to the hallway. I have a notion about this. Although most of the time he said he did not remember it, Rex was raped anally when he was 4 years old, repeatedly over several months; I think he still, unconsciously, could not tolerate anyone looking at him from behind. So, unaware but as a marker of this, he turned halfway around, waved, and said "goodbye" a second time. There was a need to interrupt me looking at him go.

~

Rex was born in the United States to two South American immigrants who had met in the United States. I never met his father; at the time I began working with Rex, his father was serving a prison sentence for selling drugs. After his release, his contact with his children was very sporadic and invariably problematic. He did not contribute to their support but would occasionally buy them expensive basketball shoes, restimulating their dreams of fatherly contact and then breaking their hearts every time.

Rex's mother, with whom I met regularly for adjunctive sessions, was the middle daughter of a middle-class family. She completed the better part of a university education in two separate fields before emigrating to the United States, in part because she saw limited prospects for herself, personally and professionally, in her own country, and in part perhaps because of stereotyped fantasies of U.S. immigrants. She was caring but equivocally attuned to her children, uneven in her skills as a parent, and quite overwhelmed by the many demands of her impoverished current lifestyle.

When Rex's parents married, they lived in a Latin slum in another state. The father would spend lengthy times away from home, leaving the mother alone and isolated in a foreign country. In retrospect, she felt she should have known that such a pattern of behavior was irregular and suspect; at the time, she did not know, or at least could not admit to herself that she knew.

Rex, the oldest of three children (two from this husband, one from another), was born into this unhappy atmosphere. During his earliest years he was witness to numerous instances of domestic violence, including one, when Rex was 2 years old, during which the father threw a pot of hot spaghetti at his wife's face. Rex is reported to have screamed at him to stop and to have come to his mother's protection. I suspect this incident is remembered because its confusing amalgam of symbolic maternal nurturance (she was cooking dinner), food, intimacy, and violence is at the core of Rex's inner experience. Historically, it may have the character of an apocryphal memory, but, like many such impressions, it preserves in crystallized form important elements of affect and experience.

The parents separated when Rex was 2 or 3, with the mother taking custody, although they never pursued a formal adjudication of their *de facto* divorce or a legal decision on custody—one of the many aspects of the family's life that, by never becoming clear, allowed fantasies to blossom and fester. A few months after the separation, according to Rex's mother—who could not tell the story straightforwardly—the father kidnapped Rex and took him to his native country, where he lived in a remote drug-processing encampment with his North American girlfriend. In the perverse logic of Rex's life, he lost his Spanish and learned English in this setting because the girlfriend, who was his caretaker, did not speak Spanish.

The mother, with the help of her extended family, went to the country and brought Rex back to the United States, where she began a life, never particularly happy or safe, as a single mother on welfare. They have lived in poor communities in Hispanic population centers in various parts of the United States ever since.

Rex's life has been filled with "accidents"; the quotation marks reflect the fact that, as these are explored, they seem anything but accidental, but rather seem determined by rich, chilling, psychodynamic meanings. When asked to tell about Rex's early life, the mother described him as loving and bright, but so active and willful that she was never able to control or supervise him as she would have wanted. What I heard in this was that, in part as a function of his own temperament and in part as a reaction to the experience of a narcissistic caregiver, Rex would simultaneously mirror the mother's narcissistic disregard, behave in extreme and self-endangering ways as a maneuver to get bits of attention and protection from her, act out his rage at her for her many deprivations, and react to his inner pain by genuinely and literally trying to destroy himself. At a young age, Rex is reported to have fallen out of a window. This may have been a kind of protest against the quality of the mother's caretaking and vigilance and a sense that the conditions of his life were hopeless, in any case worth escaping by a leap into a void.

When he was 4 years old, a boarder the mother had taken in to help pay the rent raped Rex anally repeatedly over a series of several months. The mother's ignorance of this at the time follows closely a pattern analysts have described in which a parent's problematic caregiving creates a climate in which sexual abuse is more likely (Levine, 1990). After the abuse was disclosed, Rex received several months of brief, focal psychotherapy in a special program for sexually abused children. He has no memory of this, and only the slightest trace of memory of the abuse itself; he almost never initiated a discussion about it with me. It is perhaps significant that this brief therapy was conducted in English, which Rex speaks with near-native fluency and almost no accent. However, the whole of his affective experience is encoded in Spanish, which he holds onto with a fierceness that at times can be startling. For example, when he did not know a Spanish term but did know its English equivalent, a common experience for U.S. Hispanics, he would steadfastly refuse to use the English word. My speculation is that Rex clings to Spanish as his one way of keeping connection, albeit out of consciousness, with his early traumas, which are integral to his identity and encoded for him only in Spanish.

The mother is an evangelical Christian, and church has always been an important part of her life and Rex's. (This fact will have a meaning for Latin Americans that is hard to communicate. Latin America is largely Catholic, but evangelical Protestantism has grown rapidly in recent years, often in its more extreme forms, as a response to a widespread disillusionment with what is traditional and ineffective.) One day, when he was 7, Rex heard in church a sermon on the text "if thine eye offends thee, cast it out," and went home and tried to poke out his eye. This act may have had several determinants: a means of undoing the fact that Rex had seen his rape; a defense against an ego-dystonic wish (i.e., one inconsistent with his beliefs) to suicide; a way of feeling close to God and mother—a kind of cry to them; a displacement of and punishment for a wish to poke and bite the mother, as an infant might bite a "bad breast" that did not readily yield milk; a simultaneous identification with and attack against the absent, malign, but powerful and effective father; the impulsive act of a child whose traumatization and caregiving have been such that impulse control is equivocal; an attempt at discovery and adventure. What is inescapable is that it left Rex blinded in one eye. I suspect that many children living in a violent and chaotic world become disabled in ways that are really not very dissimilar. I suspect that if we dug as deeply into the lives of many other children with disabilities in the Third World (and not just in the Third World) as it has been possible to do with Rex in the course of his analytic treatment, we would find similar horrors.

Rex received treatment for his eye wound at a prominent inner city teaching institution, simultaneously a paragon of high-tech U.S. medicine and a refuge for the many tragedies of a large city, a hectic and often confusing place. Thus, while Rex was treated by world-famous physicians and surgeons, rarely was anything explained in detail (or in Spanish) to him and his mother. The treatments were painful and frightening, and Rex would often refuse to cooperate. At one point the physicians believed that, if Rex's seeing eye were covered for several months, his injured eye might regain some of its function, but he refused. Similarly, while his physician had told him he should not play contact sports because if he injured his other eye he would be blind, he had never agreed to this, and his mother was never able to stop him from playing. Rex took a strong measure of fantasy pride from his physical ability, which was good, but he was constrained by his limited capacity to receive visual input.

At the time he began treatment with me, Rex had been seen for a couple of years by a talented bilingual clinician with limited training at a public clinic. Not surprisingly in such settings, the structure of the therapy was problematic; the therapist was often absent for meetings or long leaves. The regularity of sessions would often be affected by other reasons as well, such as giving some of Rex's time to the mother, meeting with school or other helping personnel, or making home and hospital visits to offer support and practical help. While these disruptions of a regular individual therapy schedule were well intentioned, I learned that they had deeply bothered Rex. I wondered whether the therapist's countertransference (her feelings provoked by her experience of Rex's feelings toward her and treatment of her) might have played a role, and in a conversation with her she validated this. Being with Rex was hard; breaks were a relief.

Rex's behavior both at home and at school was highly problematic. At home, he was angry, disobedient, and demanding. While he could emerge from this to be loving and sensitive, the more common alternative to rage was a frighteningly deep depressive withdrawal. Toward his younger brother, who was partially deaf, with a partial facial paralysis, slight figure, and infantile manner suggestive of psychogenic failure to thrive, he would be intensely rivalrous, consistently berating, and often dangerously violent.

Rex's school at the time was a public elementary school in one of the most impoverished parts of an otherwise affluent county, a chaotic and poorly run place in which it would be hard to imagine anyone doing well. While Rex's IQ score was originally measured in the superior range, it had slipped several notches during his time in this school. He would rarely work on task and often would stalk around the classroom, scowling and attacking others at will; there were frequent fights outside of class as well. Rex's version of this was that other children attacked him, and when he attempted to tell school authorities about it they ignored him. Indeed, many of his classmates were violent children, and I directly observed many instances when the school was flagrantly unresponsive.

Rex was in a self-contained class for children with emotional/behavioral disorders, run on a strict behavior modification program. This was a source of constant frustration to Rex, because he could never achieve enough "points" to gain any measure of socially validated success. The dynamics of his traumatization and the equivocal nature of his emotional and behavioral control were such that, even when he was trying his best, he could not have very many "good days." When the school felt Rex had done something particularly grievous, or when he was simply beyond their control, they would call his mother. She felt humiliated by the constant phone calls (in English, which she did not speak or understand well) and was no more capable of dealing with Rex than the school was.

As Rex progressed in therapy, he started to improve in school. His underlying brightness came out when the teachers began to have better expectations of him and challenged him more. Positive feedback for his improved academic performance led to better behavior. He was switched to a regular fifth-grade class and did well.

Then a tragedy occurred. When Rex moved on to middle school, he was accompanied by papers that stated he was a special education student but omitted to mention that he had been returned to a regular class. Rex was placed in special education classes again, except this time on a middle-school level, with bigger, scarier, more violent kids, and teachers who had less patience and nurturance. Rex had a terrible fall, and neither his mother nor I could figure out why. He felt afraid all the time, went back to saying no one believed him or understood him, and began getting very aggressive. One day he blurted out to me that we had all lied to him, that we had been telling him he was in regular classes and then put him back into special classes. That was the first time his mother and I realized what had happened. Rex was put back into regular classes, but in the remaining 2 years of my work with him, his behavior and achievement in school continued to deteriorate. Perhaps the inadvertent switch back to special classes was complicated by the beginning hormonal changes of puberty or the increased social stressors of middle school.

One summer I wangled Rex's admission into a summer camp for emotionally disturbed kids. He loved the experience—the free T-shirt, being a member of a group with a name, going swimming (Rex's mother rarely took him anywhere)—and began to blossom socially. He made some friends. Another summer the mother got her family to pay for plane tickets and took Rex and his brother and sister for a 6-week visit to her native country. Again, Rex thrived. Economics were not so tight because the extended family paid for everything. There was household help and plenty of food. Rex could play soccer in a park across the street; there were no safe parks where his family lived in the United States. The depression and aggressiveness faded. So there was something in Rex that could function with pleasure and effectiveness, in the right environment.

But then it was time to come home—to no money, no safe neighborhood, certainly no servants, no outings, and the same school where Rex was convinced he was hated. His grades were poor; homework did not get done; and there were frequent aggressive episodes. The mother continued to be overwhelmed by her life circumstances and by her own psychological issues.

By this point the mother had had it. She could not control Rex and was sick of trying. She resisted accepting that she had any role in his behavior, although it seemed clear this was part of the problem. There was a direct correlation between the amount of attention she gave Rex and his behavior. When she locked herself in her room for hours on end, would not speak to Rex, and would not intervene when his brother called him names and hit him, Rex became aggressive and depressed. When she sat with him during homework, found 20 minutes to talk to him about his day, and praised him for the positive things he did, his hope returned and his fists went down.

But she ignored this reality and soon stopped spending special time with Rex. She signed up for college courses—a positive move in her life, but one that she used as a reason for withdrawing her time and attention from Rex. Objectively, she could have found 20 minutes a day for Rex even with her studies, but she did not. She stopped seeing me regularly. Although I told her I thought Rex would not improve without her regular sessions with me, I did not refuse to continue seeing him.

Rex's mother began being absent from the house for many hours a day; when she was home, she spent hours in her bedroom doing homework, while Rex and his siblings ran around screaming and hitting each other. I had a hard time seeing this as solely Rex's fault, although I did not hesitate to confront him about his own contributions to the situation. I tried to be diplomatic and walk the tightropes with Rex (they should not hit you; you should not hit them) and his mother (I am glad you are making a life for yourself; your children need you). I was empathic with both parties, sympathizing with the mother's need for a break and Rex's need for his mother. But this approach did not work. Conflict at home escalated.

Rex's middle school was not supportive of the therapy. They felt a behavior modification approach would be more effective. I pointed out they were doing behavior modification with him competently, and its impact seemed limited. I felt our efforts could be complementary, but we never succeeded in meshing as a team.

As things got worse, the school felt Rex should be hospitalized. I was not averse to this idea, but no local hospitals would accept Rex as a patient without major advocacy efforts because they did not accept Medical Assistance, the public insurance the family had. However, the mother oscillated: more than once, she would ask me to hospitalize Rex, but when I would make the arrangements—which took many unpaid hours—she would change her mind.

Things were in a state of constant crisis when Rex disappeared. I got a call on my answering machine from the mother that he would be away for a week. For the next 2 months, I tried unsuccessfully to reach Rex and his mother but there were no answers to my phone calls at their home. I was frustrated but also had to admit I was relieved. I wondered whether something in the unconscious life of Rex or his mother or some error I had made in therapy had driven them away. Perhaps this outcome should just be attributed to the chaos in life of poor people. And then, after a while, I stopped wondering.

Some time later Rex's mother called me and announced they had been in South America and were back. She asked if I could see Rex the next day, assuming I would. When I told her the hours were filled, she asked if I could see him the day after. It took a while for her to understand that my waiting list at that time was months long. My work with Rex was over.

~

I still cannot think about my work with Rex without intense disquiet. I know that there were deep, healing moments in this therapy.

Rex came to feel that his most primitive and powerful elements of intolerable experience were successfully projected, contained, and undergoing a process of transformation. There were times when he came out of his shell, advanced in his self-esteem, learned actively, and began to feel that a decent life was possible for him. I am aware that these are significant accomplishments, hard-won for both Rex and me. Many complex dynamics became clear to me through my work with Rex, and I have memories of tender and powerful therapeutic moments with him. Some of these lessons surface when I am now able to do with other children with disabilities what I was unable to do before.

And yet the therapy did not achieve its goals. Neither Rex nor his mother reached enough insight or motivation to fundamentally overcome their problems. Perhaps both have enough biologically based mental illness and too few concrete resources and social supports to achieve a good outcome. Or perhaps Rex's trauma was just too severe and destroyed his mind and his heart the way it destroyed his eye.

I do not blame others who tried to help Rex and saw things differently from me. Many good people have worked very hard to try to help Rex and his family. All of us have felt our task may well have been impossible, beyond the reach of our abilities and efforts. I also do not blame Rex's mother in any way; I see her as a woman whose difficult circumstances made it hard for her to work out her own issues. Maybe I believed in a very dangerous fantasy that therapy would fix what it can never, or almost never, fix.

One of the things I learned, or relearned, through my work with Rex is that many people with disabilities really do live desperate, empty lives. Some of this is because of disability issues, some because of other life circumstances. Are such people beyond the reach of psychotherapy? I do not suspect Rex's situation is uncommon, except in the sense that he somehow found his way to spending several years with a therapist who really loved him and worked hard to try to help him. And I wonder how the unhealed pain of all those other Rexes keeps from exploding, and what will happen when it eventually does.

REFERENCE

Levine, H. (Ed.). (1990). *Adult analysis and childhood sexual abuse.* Hillsdale, NJ: Analytic Press.

4

Matthew

Therapy with a Teenager with a Disability

Rhoda Olkin

Therapy with teenagers, like teenagers themselves, tends to be intense, but also rich with possibilities for growth and development. This case, of a 14-year old boy with mild cerebral palsy, illustrates how the issue of the client's disability and the need to understand disability issues in a developmental context pervade therapy. This chapter presents the case chronologically, pausing periodically to comment on the disability issues as they arose.

The therapy itself was brief, encompassing only three sessions with the teenager himself. But this belies the complexity of the therapeutic involvement, which included over 5 hours of phone contact plus two sessions with the parents, consultations with the parents' therapist, a referral for a neuropsychological battery, approximately 2 hours of phone time with school personnel and referral possibilities, and hours spent reading developmental and assessment reports encompassing the time since the client was 7 months old. I also read a chapter on cerebral palsy for my own education (Stolov & Clowers, 1981, which follows a medical model, but has useful information about physical and cognitive aspects of various disabilities). I consider such review a necessary first step for any therapist working with a client with a disability—to understand the general parameters of a disability and then to learn the particulars from the client.

~

Matthew, a 14-year-old boy with cerebral palsy, was referred to me in private practice by another therapist who had been working with Matthew's parents in couples' therapy for a few months. The parents had mentioned their only child and his disability, a mild cerebral palsy affecting predominantly one side. They seemed concerned about his welfare, although there was no specific presenting problem.

Two issues were already apparent. First, although we are often aware of the paucity of role models for people with disabilities, this same issue also affects parents of a child with a disability. They, too, lack role models for 1) comparison with other children of their child's behaviors and development, 2) their own parenting as it interacts with the disability, 3) expected age-appropriate developmental stages, and 4) expected outcomes for their child as an adult. It was premature to know if their concerns merely required reassurance or signaled more troubling developmental or emotional difficulties in the child.

Second, the therapist seeing the parents had the foresight to recommend a therapist with expertise in disability, and one who had a disability herself. The inclination might have been to seek someone more expert with teenagers, but the referring therapist, whom I will call Dr. D, felt the disability issues would be paramount. However, the referral was tricky; the parents, whom I call Mr. and Mrs. Y, were not ready to admit disability as a dominant issue for their son.

Dr. D managed the delicate issue of the referral, suggested that the parents call me, and alerted me to the possibility. Mrs. Y then called me. I had already decided to spend more than the usual amount of time with her during this first call. Thus, we initially spoke for about 45 minutes, during which I helped her figure out how to present the idea of therapy to her son, broached the subject of her son's disability openly, revealed my own disability without supplying details, and began to lay the groundwork for elevating the issue of disability to greater prominence. I suggested that Matthew would need to come to his own understanding of his disability, separately from his parents, and that this might need to occur in a milieu outside the familial arena. A second phone call confirmed the appointment and reiterated some of what had already transpired in the first call. Matthew had agreed to the suggested three sessions.

I decided to spend this telephone time with Mrs. Y because I felt it was usual and appropriate for the mother of a child with a disability to be vigilant in prescreening medical, school, and other professionals before subjecting her son to incursions on his life. Thus I surmised that she was unlikely to bring Matthew to see me until *she* felt comfortable with me. This should not be construed as an "overinvolved" mother.

Matthew arrived with his mother for the first session and was hesitant to separate from her. I shook Mrs. Y's hand but did not extend my hand to Matthew, whose right side was the one affected. As she started to leave, he joked that he'd rap on the window if he needed rescuing. In other ways his behavior was reminiscent of an 8- to 9-year old. He sometimes acted as if things could be made to go away—by "not remembering" or, when he didn't like my questions (usually directly about disability), swiveling his chair 180 degrees and speaking with his back to me. He'd comment on things in my office rather than answer anxiety-provoking questions. He sometimes contradicted himself, and when I pointed out some of these instances he was untroubled by the disparities. Yet in other ways his understanding was at least at a 14-year-old level, and his vocabulary was excellent. For example, I started to say that something was paradoxical, and he finished the thought: that on the one hand he "likes being disabled," yet he tries to hide it.

Matthew tried to portray the image of someone comfortable with his disability, but his behavior, and occasionally his words, betrayed him. He commented favorably on my not extending my hand to him; that is a situation he tries to avoid. He could name at least 10 friends, yet he rarely got phone calls and all his weekend activities were spent with his parents. He spoke of lying to adults about the reason for his disability, telling outrageous (and viscerally evocative) lies, such as being run over by a bus. He felt responsible for his parents being in therapy, sensing that his disability was a problem for them, at least financially; however, he made clear he didn't want to know if this was the case, because he couldn't handle the answer. He also raised the subject of suicide, but denied current suicidal ideation. He did not tell me, as his mother had, that he had threatened suicide the previous summer.

I considered possible *DSM-IV* (American Psychiatric Association, 1994) diagnoses after the first session. I felt that Pervasive Developmental Disorder (PDD) was too severe, especially given Matthew's understanding of my comments and questions, his own use of language to communicate ideas, and his keen desire for friends and acceptance by peers. His swiveling in his chair, while reminiscent of PDD, was more likely simply avoidance, especially given the clear link between our conversation and his behavior. I considered depression, which manifests differently for adolescents than for adults, and felt it was premature to either include or preclude this diagnosis. A probable diagnosis was Academic Skills Disorders (specifically Developmental Arithmetic and Expressive Writing Disorders). These are precluded by a neurological disorder, but I didn't have sufficient information to address that. Axis III noted the hemiplegia affecting the right side of the body—including arm, hand, leg, foot—and left side of the brain.

The problem of diagnosis raised the question of a model for intervention. I subscribe wholeheartedly to a minority model of disability, yet the diagnoses available are based on a medical model and clearly place the pathology within the individual. There is no diagnosis that says, "I'm counter to society's expectations and having a hard time of it."

It was important for Matthew, even in the context of meeting someone else with a disability, to be seen as "normal" or at least not to emphasize his disability initially (and he therefore appreciated not having to shake my hand). Thus, we had begun walking the precarious line between addressing the proverbial elephant in the room and respecting Matthew's defenses and control over his own presentation. This line began to feel thinner after Matthew's next behaviors.

I received a phone call from Dr. D to let me know that both Mr. and Mrs. Y had (separately) called him, very upset about Matthew's report of our session. Matthew had told his parents that I asked if he felt like committing suicide, asked about a particular method, and when he didn't know about this method explained to him how it worked; that I asked, "Do you have a problem with that?" in response to his question about our (shared) religion; and that I implied that it was Matthew's fault that his parents were in therapy. Dr. D had reassured the parents that this did not sound like me and encouraged them to call me directly.

That afternoon Mrs. Y called me and raised these issues. I responded to her concerns, going through each one and giving a context and my wording. For example, I said that I would routinely assess suicide potential in a 14-year-old, and, had it not come up, I would have brought it up at some point (though perhaps not in an initial session). However, Matthew was the first to mention it, referring to "going suicidal" if he heard information he couldn't handle. Some of Matthew's allegations were distortions of conversations; others were complete fabrications.

It was clear that Mrs. Y wanted to believe me, but this put her in a dilemma. It forced her to ask herself why Matthew would lie, which she felt was out of character for him, and, even more worrisome, why he would bring up suicide. I responded during this call with basic Rogerian congruence (i.e., behavior that is congruent with one's true feelings). When she asked how I'd felt when I'd heard these allegations from Dr. D, I replied truthfully that I was very surprised and upset to hear anyone say I would do these things, which were quite unprofessional. I was also very empathetic with her position of having to face new and disturbing information about Matthew. Then, after about 45 minutes, I asked her to have faith in her own perceptions of me. I hoped that after spending some amount of time on the phone with me (on three occasions) that she trusted herself to make a judgment about me. This seemed to convince her. She alluded to Matthew sometimes behaving in ways that were "immature and inappropriate." I had not known if she was aware of this, since no information about any developmental delays or cognitive impairments had been discussed with her up to this point. Her raising the topic allowed me to inquire about any developmental delays, which she confirmed, and to request copies of school tests (which she agreed to send me). She confirmed that Matthew would keep his next appointment. She called back shortly afterwards to report that Matthew had essentially admitted to lying.

Mr. Y called a few days later. He seemed to have accepted Mrs. Y's report of her conversation with me and was therefore concerned about Matthew's potential for suicide and whether it was safe to leave Matthew home alone for an evening. He also wondered about the potential for therapy to "burst Matthew's bubble" that he is okay in the world, that his disability is accepted, and that he can be what he wants to be. Mr. Y mentioned that Matthew wanted to try out for the football team and that he (the father) didn't want to tell him no. He asked how long therapy would be; I repeated the three-session agreement, after which I would meet with the parents.

After only one session with Matthew, I did not feel I knew him well. Yet I was compelled to defend my professional integrity, make judgments about suicide potential, reassure understandably alarmed parents, and respond to specific questions about football, length of therapy, and so forth. Even more, I needed to begin to understand Matthew's behavior toward me and decide on a stance for the next session. My initial response was to the inherent hostility of Matthew's actions. It discredited me and gave him a way to avoid returning. I viewed this lying to his parents as conceptually related to his lying to other adults about the cause of his disability. Both struck me as angry acts. This was significant because nothing in Matthew's overt presentation or in his mother's description of him even touched on anger. The requirement for regulation of affect is strong for people with disabilities (Olkin, 1993). In general, there is a prescription for pluckiness and courage and a prohibition against anger. Perhaps Matthew had internalized this and only displayed his anger in limited arenas. Perhaps too his parents were slow to recognize his anger, out of their own desire to view him as coping with his disability. Furthermore, he may have felt that his anger could not be directed at them, but only toward safer targets; they were his safety net, and he couldn't afford to alienate them.

But before I could interpret the anger, it was important to ask whether I should think about this behavior in light of Matthew's chronological age or a possibly developmentally delayed emotional age. The latter led me to speculate that this was not so much anger as a testing of boundaries and limits, reminiscent of younger children trying to figure out who will know what (i.e., will my mother know if I'm naughty in school?). In this case, Matthew probably wanted to know what his parents would know about the therapy session and whether he could control the information.

~

For the second session, Matthew came into my waiting room alone. His behavior in this session was much more attentive. Although he swiveled in his chair, he kept it facing me, never turning his back. Having decided to be straightforward but nonjudgmental, I began by discussing our last session, letting him know of his parents' phone calls. He wasn't surprised that his mother called and said, "She always calls; they look out for me." But he was surprised that she called twice and that his father also had called, indicating that a call from dad meant trouble (for me). In reviewing the first session, he genuinely seemed to believe much of what he had alleged had taken place. Since there was little point in getting into an I-said/you-said debate, I dropped it. Instead, I focused on whether Matthew did not want to be in therapy and therefore may have been trying to discredit me. He quickly got the connection. In a roundabout way he asserted he liked coming to see me, although he called it "a hassle."

I told Matthew the gist of the preschool and school reports I'd read. I gave him some compliments (for which he seemed hungry) and acknowledged his difficulties in some areas (math and written language). I said he had a kind of learning disability (LD), but that it had nothing to do with intelligence. Although he said, "I know that," he added, "I guess I'll never go to Harvard." I responded, "Why not? Lots of my graduate students have LD."

Once we got over the hurdle of Matthew's beginning relationship with me, I began the work of therapy, which included assessing his understanding of and feelings about his disability. I didn't want to make any assumptions about what he had been told or understood about his disability and its meaning and implications. This was especially important given his age, but I have found that even older adults with disabilities carry misconceptions and myths about their disability from childhood.

Matthew talked about his "inner and outer self" (his distinction). He described his inner self in positive terms. His outer self was described more neutrally (height, weight, eye and hair color), and he hedged about whether he had a disability. When asked about his goals for therapy, he immediately said that he'd like his right side to be like his left side. He alluded to becoming frustrated and angry about having to work so hard at school just to keep up. He reported punching file cabinets and walls when he got angry. When I teased him about taking care of his "good" hand, he responded to the humor without taking offense. At the end of the session, I brought his mother in from the waiting room to request permission to talk with the resource specialist; both Matthew and his mother signed the release form.

Matthew, like many people with disabilities, had internalized the negative messages about disability and had divided himself into his inner and outer selves. From the perspective of his internal experience he was free of his body, without disabilities, and replete with positive attributes. However, he was also aware of others' responses to him and to his disability. This physical outer self reflected the perceptions of outsiders. This duality led to an uncomfortable coexistence, a split self-concept that was not yet reconciled. Such a split could lead to cognitive dissonance at the least, and perhaps more severe symptoms. In Matthew they led to a sense of unease in his own body, an inchoate anger that erupted sporadically, and occasional lying to protect his disabled identity. A goal for treatment (or for Matthew on his own) would need to include a reconciliation between these two selves—an incorporation of his disability into his self-concept, without the concomitant incorporation of society's negative messages about the disability.

As a minor, Matthew did not have to give permission for me to speak with his resource teacher. However, I included him in the discussion and actually had him sign the release form for two reasons. First, as a more general therapeutic issue with a 14-year-old, self-determination and control can be prominent issues, and therefore it is appropriate to keep the teenager abreast of all aspects of intervention. Second, it was particularly important for Matthew because a key therapeutic goal was to give him increasing ownership of his disability. This included receiving information, making decisions, and developing his own feelings and stance about it. Throughout the therapy I wanted to remain true to this goal.

Shortly thereafter I had a phone consult with Matthew's resource teacher, Ms. R, with whom Matthew spends two periods per day. She confirmed much of the written reports from various testing done over the years. She also was very informative about Matthew's social development and her responses to him. Her fondness for him was evident, as was her worry for him. She was particularly concerned about his transition from middle to high school the following year and his desire to fit in with the football crowd. She noted that, although improved, he was still impulsive in his work, rushing through things, and less mature than others his age. She remarked on his "silly" jokes; he could still "get a laugh" out of the other kids, but the jokes were increasingly "inappropriate" as other kids matured. She commented on his seeking of adult attention over that of his peers; she felt that adults were "safer" for him. She said that she and Matthew never discussed his disability directly, only its manifestations (e.g., learning difficulties), and she gave examples of how she'd helped him with his work. She concurred with Mrs. Y that Matthew didn't really have any friends and said she'd tried unsuccessfully to have him connect with other boys in the resource room. She said that he's "not teased, kids are kind to him," but he's on the fringe, "tolerated."

I wanted to understand Matthew in the context of his age, development, school tasks, and social arena. Matthew could not be the sole source for information in these areas, and resource teachers are often the school personnel who know kids with disabilities the best. Thus Ms. R was able to fill in some specific gaps (e.g., about the types of learning difficulties Matthew experiences). But her personal responses to Matthew were also invaluable. My impression was that she was very fond of him, perhaps more so than other kids under her tutelage. She went out of her way to help him, sometimes more than she should. She felt hope for his more distant future but concern for his more immediate experiences as an adolescent. She was an important relationship for Matthew and would be a significant loss for him when he moved on to high school. Thus, her countertransference with Matthew (i.e., her own responses to Matthew, based on both her own history and psychological makeup, as well as those aspects of Matthew manifest in her relationship with him) in some ways mirrored my own. Despite what he'd put me through after the initial visit, I too felt fond of him and eager to help him. Her responses also alerted me to behaviors on my part to avoid, namely doing more for him than I should. Furthermore, if I was going to be a different kind of relationship for him, one way would be for me to be one of the few (and possibly the only) adult who spoke with him directly about his disability. Lastly, some of the things Ms. R told me about Matthew's social situation broke my heart: how he was a football player wanna-be, hanging onto the fringe, tolerated but not a part of the group. She implied what I had felt, that his adolescence might be a more-than-usually painful experience and that although he would emerge okay the going would be rough.

The talk with Ms. R had another value. She and I agreed on desired directions to work on with Matthew. We decided to focus on two of these. The first was to increase his competence and comfort with computers; we both felt that he could learn to do some of the tasks on the computer that presently required help from a resource specialist. If he could do them on computer, it would increase his independence. The second was to try to direct Matthew's social interest into a wider arena, beyond (but not precluding) football. Our agreement meant that Matthew would be getting consistent messages from two important sources. This is vital when working with children and adolescents.

~

For the third session Matthew again came in by himself. I asked him if he'd like to try my (electric three-wheeled) scooter at the end of the session; he seemed eager and pleased about this. This proved to be a good reinforcer, because I forced Matthew to stick to uncomfortable topics longer than he wanted. I asked him about trying out for freshman football the next fall, which he adamantly confirmed. I told him point-blank that I thought it was a bad idea, and why: that he would continue to experience increasing discrepancies between his own athletic abilities and those of his peers, that I was afraid he'd be on the bench for the year, never really a "part of the team," but a "hanger-on." However, I also said that this was my opinion and that the decision was his. He surprised me by asking about whether it was wrong to strive for something.

Matthew's question is a central one in disability. What is the distinction between knowing and respecting your realistic limits, and giving up or using the disability as an excuse? How do you simultaneously strive to be and do your best, and accept your own limitations without fighting them and denying your disability? In Matthew's case, was trying out for freshman football a realistic striving, or yielding to the message to be an "overcomer"—that is, to "overcome" the disability by being as much like everyone else as possible. The answer is that there is no answer; in each instance, it is hard to tell the difference. One can only look at the pattern.

I wondered if Matthew knew the story of his birth (and onset of his disability). He partly did and was able to cite a reason for his disability, but further probing found that he was unable to go beyond the usual one-to-two sentence response. He said he'd be afraid to know the full story. This theme of not wanting to know more came up several more times: He didn't want to talk about the disability, to hear his parents' opinion about his trying out for football, to know why his parents were in therapy, to hear the story of his birth. Most emphatically he did not want to come to a session with his parents. At times he seemed close to tears. Overall he was much more serious, although he was increasingly sarcastic as I stayed with these topics. Finally he told me, "You have 2 more minutes" (to finish up this topic), and he set the timer on his watch. I used the 2 minutes to have him repeat back the messages he'd heard from me so I could correct any distortions. Then I respected the time limit. At one point I found myself calling him "hon," much like I do my own children, as if in response to his underlying fear. I reminded him I'd be meeting with his parents next time and told him what I'd be recommending to them. This included a neuropsychological exam and a left-handed keyboard for the computer. He had gotten wind of the request for a neuropsychological evaluation and had some questions about it (which, interestingly, he asked me rather than his mother). I answered them and went beyond his questions to unasked ones. I assured him it was a noninvasive procedure and would not hurt in any way, and I gave him information on the tasks involved and how long it would take.

At the end of the session, I did not push for any closure on whether he would continue to see me. I reminded him of the three-session limit and asked him to let me know himself of his decision (not to have his parents tell me). Then, as promised, I gave him a brief lesson on how to ride my scooter (using his left hand only), and he rode it down the hallway, through the lobby, and back again.

By this third session, it had become increasingly apparent that Matthew's disability was a major factor in his present functioning and emotional state. He seemed to spend a great deal of psychic and emotional energy responding to his disability. He had to work extra hard at all his school tasks and assignments. He was trying to fit in a social milieu where physical prowess was esteemed and rewarded. He tried to hide his disability from people he didn't know. He lacked any role models for disability, and he was acutely aware of the other few students at his school with disabilities and their lower status. He was afraid to discuss his disability, to learn more about it, to try to work *with* it rather than *around* it. And underneath it all was a scared boy who tried to be the class clown, but who often felt depressed, angry, and scared, even suicidal.

My desire to know what Matthew knew about his disability was part of my goal of increasing his ownership of and responsibility for his condition. The story of the disability should be *his* story, but at that time it was still his parents' story, and one he hadn't even fully heard. Parents (and other adults) often erroneously believe that their child has heard the full story before and that he or she understands it. For example, parents may say, "We've told him about his disability," but they may have told him at an early age and not updated the facts to accommodate increasing maturity and ability to understand. They may also have assumed understanding without verifying it. I saw as a necessary first step having his parents tell Matthew the full story of his birth, making sure he understood and giving him a chance to ask questions. I also wanted them to tell him not just the facts, but their responses to those facts: their feelings about his disability and their struggles with it. This is necessary because I believe he picked up on this anyway, but because it wasn't "on the table," he was not free to ask or comment about it. Also, if Matthew was to come to his own understanding of his disability, he first needed to hear and discuss his parents' responses, and especially the ways in which his parents did and did not agree with each other about it. This would open the possibility for Matthew to formulate his own responses.

After Matthew's third session I met with his parents. I had a list of things I wanted to cover in my meeting with the parents, which included getting to know them and their feelings about and perspectives on Matthew and his disability. They also wanted to discuss the freshman football issue (Matthew had led me to believe that they had signed the requisite forms and were willing to let him try out for the team).

Although persons with disabilities are referred to as a minority group, their status is unlike other minority groups (except gays and lesbians) in that they are usually the only one with that minority status in the family. Thus the primary source of support—the family—that is available for other minority groups is absent for those with disabilities. Furthermore (again, like gays and lesbians), not only might the family not be a source of support, but they can be part of the problem. Their attitudes toward the minority condition may contain much of the same prejudices as society's. Therefore, to assess Matthew meant likewise assessing his parents and their responses to his disability—not only how they felt about it, but their hopes and fears for him, how they talk to him about it, and what they think he can and cannot do.

Mr. and Mrs. Y relayed the story of Matthew's birth, which had been life-threatening for Mrs. Y. I asked some questions that they couldn't answer. We reviewed their discovery of Matthew's disability (at around 7 months) and their subsequent search for a diagnosis and assistance. After a flurry of activity in Matthew's first 6 years or so (physical therapy, occupational therapy, testing, consultations, school placements, and so forth) they seemed to have settled into a pattern around his disability. Mother was active in seeking information and school- and doctor-related questions; Father was her supportive backup and made follow-up calls as needed. They discussed Matthew's disability with him matter-of-factly, focusing on the physical and learning aspects to the exclusion of the emotional and psychosocial factors. They were scared of what I was going to say to them, prepared to hear that their view of their son was somehow "wrong" and that they had missed vital clues to his psychological status.

In discussing the football question, they let me know that they were not prepared for Matthew to play football, but their primary reason (physical safety) was different than mine (psychological well-being). The important thing, I felt, was that Matthew be given the information, then allowed to make his own decision.

I recommended a neuropsychological evaluation. I explained that up until now Matthew's disability had been evaluated predominantly as it affected his body and his learning. However, it had not told us about Matthew as a person. It treated him as a "part object," and it was time to put the whole together. Entering adolescence was a precipitant for this need. They readily agreed to the evaluation.

I had several other suggestions for them. First, I had investigated computer modifications that allowed using the keyboard entirely left-handed and discovered that IBM supplied this software for free. I gave them a rationale for increasing Matthew's comfort with computers and for doing so in a way that didn't highlight his disability (as two-handed keyboards seemed to do for him) and that maximized his independence. Second, I recommended a book for Matthew, but suggested they read some of it first (Kriegsman, Zaslow, & D'Zmura-Rechsteiner, 1992). Third, I gave them a reference for a recording of a left-handed only classical pianist. Last, I recommended they hold a family meeting to tell Matthew the story of his disability. In response to their question, I suggested they not push Matthew to make a decision about seeing me beyond the three sessions. He did not seem ready to decide, and there was no urgency. We concluded by setting up a second appointment for the parents in 2 weeks.

Many parents come to therapy expecting to be blamed for their children's problems, and of course it's important that this not occur. Therefore, when I met with Matthew's parents, I started with a compliment on how well they were raising their son. I framed my suggestions as improvements for an already solid base. However, I did suggest, in many ways and guises, that the issue of disability was more paramount than they acknowledged, and I tried to convey the difficulties of being a teenager with a physical and learning disability. Most particularly, I wanted to move our discussion from Matthew's physical and learning disability to the psychosocial aspects of being a person with a disability. Too often people with disabilities are treated as part objects by physicians, teachers, school psychologists, and physical therapists. They are tested for academic deficits, learning problems, and grade level. But Matthew was a total person, and he got lost behind the labels and descriptions of specific deficits. His emotions about his disability needed to be discussed at least as much as the mechanics.

My discussion with his parents about football exemplified this split. While they focused first on his physical safety and concerns about his hurting his "good" hand, I felt that while any physical insults could be overcome the emotional risk was great. Fortunately, the discussion about a neuropsychological evaluation helped bridge the gap; they clearly understood the need to see Matthew as a gestalt, a whole person. This was reinforced in the second session with them.

In the second session with the parents it became clear that they had done an impressive amount of thinking and talking about the issues we'd discussed in the first session. Mrs. Y put it this way: "If we can't come to grips with Matthew's disability, how can he?" They were beginning to try to come to grips with it by facing their own denial of his disability (e.g., always ending the description of him by adding, "But he's quite functional"). Furthermore, they listened carefully to my characterization of disability as a minority group and as a predominantly psychosocial experience.

They had twice tried to talk with Matthew about his birth, and both times he had clearly put them off. They had looked into left-handed keyboards and software. Mrs. Y had ordered the book on teenagers we'd discussed. They had also made a first appointment with the neuropsychologist. In short, there was a sense of movement and willingness to plunge into whatever needed to be done.

One area was especially hard for them. Matthew had no friends, and efforts they had made to help him make friends hadn't improved the situation. They described hearing him on the phone calling several people to go to a movie, being rejected each time, while they were in the next room with their hearts breaking. Tellingly, they said nothing to Matthew about this, either because they were "respecting his privacy" (dad) or unable to find the words to use (mom). Therefore an important emotional aspect of Matthew's disability had gone unspoken. I made an even stronger case than before that these were the very issues that Matthew needed help with, that had to be vocalized. They came to agree with the need, but feared the task.

We ended with an agreement for at least one more meeting. Matthew's position on therapy was still up in the air, and I again urged them not to push yet. I sensed he wanted to see what direction I seemed to be taking his parents before deciding further about me.

~

Looking back on my therapy with Matthew and his family, several issues emerged as key therapeutic cornerstones. First, a shift in perspective toward disability was called for. Up to this point Matthew had interacted with his disability as a deficit. In this mostly medical model, the onus for accommodation was on him. He had to work harder to achieve the same results as others and had to endure greater fatigue. I wanted to begin to shift the model to place greater emphasis on "reasonable accommodations" incumbent on others or in his environment. While not denouncing the value of hard work, I wanted to explore ways to make Matthew's life easier. Disability usually incurs extra work (dealing with pain and fatigue; managing one's interpersonal presentation; responding to others' questions, comments, and outright prejudices) and this, in addition to the usual turmoil of adolescence, seemed to be a heavy load for Matthew. Rather than helping him achieve his potential, I wondered if he wasn't running hard just to keep in place.

Second, it was increasingly clear that having a therapist with a disability was important not just for Matthew, but for his parents. It gave me credibility to them. Even more, the parents saw me as a powerful role model for what their son could become—successful in a career, married with children. But they also saw a large discrepancy between his present functioning and mine. I alluded to my own struggles at age 14, but in a way this was not reassuring to the parents. It took me years to come to grips with my own disability. They did not want it to take years for their son. There was a sense of urgency—to do, to help, to figure out, to answer, quickly. I found myself wanting to give them a "disability consciousness" and may have overwhelmed them in the initial session in my desire to put forth information.

Third, countertransference issues were a powerful force in this therapy. I felt an enormous affinity for Matthew. This persisted despite some very difficult behaviors on his part. I felt I understood his world from the inside, and the danger, of course, was that I might read too much of my own adolescence into his. I felt the pain he barely acknowledged and wished I could save him from it. Of course, in this I mirrored his parents' response to him. To be another adult to do this would be a mistake. As I told them, it was *his* disability; it was a lesson I had to remember myself.

The last countertransference issue was the most personally difficult. As I had the chance to help Matthew's parents see disability in a new way—as that of a disadvantaged minority group, as a predominantly psychosocial experience, as a key part of one's self-identity—I found myself reevaluating my parents, who never seemed to have "gotten" it. The more I helped Mr. and Mrs. Y do it "right," the more I saw that my own parents never would. Yet somehow, despite their limitations, I came to peace with my own disability. This, ultimately, was what I had to remember in this therapy. The journey to disability consciousness can be long and I couldn't take him to the end of the road, but I could set him on the right course.

REFERENCES

American Psychiatric Association. (1994). *Diagnostic and statistical manual of mental disorders* (4th ed.). Washington, DC: Author.

Kriegsman, K.H., Zaslow, E.L., & D'Zmura-Rechsteiner, J. (1992). *Taking charge: Teenagers talk about life and physical disabilities*. Rockville, MD: Woodbine House.

Olkin, R. (1993). Crips, gimps and epileptics explain it all to you. *Readings, 8*(4), 13–17.

Stolov, W.C., & Clowers, M.R. (Eds.). (1981). *Handbook of severe disability*. Washington, DC: U.S. Department of Education.

5

Wendy

Emerging from Behind the Mask

Mary Ann Blotzer

Wendy came with a reputation. She'd been seen at our agency before. Even our office staff, who consistently showed great patience and genuine fondness for even the quirkiest of our patients, found Wendy hard to tolerate. She evoked annoyance and sometimes condescension in them. Perhaps it was her persistent telephone calls—sometimes several within an hour—wanting to confirm the time of her appointment with me, or to change it, or to say that she didn't think she'd come that day because the weather was bad. She had a demanding, insistent quality that made others feel pestered, and there was something about her that evoked condescension from even the most respectful of persons.

The most striking characteristic about Wendy and what first telegraphs an impression of her as someone different is her voice. It's an artificial-sounding voice, not artificial in the sense of sounding mechanical, but artificial in that it comes across as an artifice, a mask that hides any clues about what she might be feeling. It's a childlike voice with little intonation, and with a strong ingratiating quality that is actually quite irritating. (Significantly, I write "it" when referring to the voice, rather than simply referring to "her voice"—more on this later.) It is as though her intent is to placate and please people, but instead of pleasing people, the underlying dynamic that fuels this mask of a voice seeps out, evoking more negative than positive reactions.

I am indebted to Rachel Ritvo, M.D., for her insightful comments on earlier drafts.

What is also significant is that Wendy's monotone is perceived as a mask. When individuals who are truly flat of affect speak in a monotone, we perceive them as congruent: the flat voice matches the flat affect. With Wendy, one senses a dissonance. That dissonance powerfully expresses a key dynamic issue of Wendy's: the tight lid she keeps on her emotions. Because her relationships are tenuous, including her own internal representations of important figures, she dares not admit negative affects into awareness. To do so would jeopardize both relationships in real time as well as her capacity to hold on to these mental representations.

Wendy's voice, with its childlike quality that makes her seem much younger than her 55 years, also reflects her accommodation to her mild mental retardation. Now that I have been seeing Wendy for 2 years, I have seen subtle shifts in her voice. During those occasions together when she has been able to tolerate greater awareness of herself and her feelings, her voice has actually sounded more authentic. And her voice is most exaggerated whenever she must deal with a new person, for example, when she calls for a cab to pick her up at the end of an appointment. On these occasions, Wendy puts on her "retarded" voice. It is as though she deliberately exaggerates her difference so that she can experience some control over it. In addition to her sense of control (since she couldn't control being born with mental retardation, she can at least control how she manifests it), another benefit is that people will see her as less capable, lower their expectations, and perhaps be more helpful to her. Because Wendy doesn't have much confidence in her effectiveness in the world (she, in fact, has a pervasive underlying sense of terror), she has developed both a personal presentation and strategies designed to get people to help her. Her underlying terror, coupled with her rigid use of this strategy, has kept her from mastering new experiences that would contribute to a greater sense of personal efficacy. Wendy keeps herself in the closet in more ways than one. Not only does she mask herself, but she assiduously avoids any new situation.

~

Wendy was referred to me by her psychiatrist, Dr. Z, who sees her once every 2 months for medication management. Wendy has been in therapy off and on since adolescence, when she had her first "breakdown." On several occasions she had been hospitalized because she had deteriorated to an actively psychotic, disorganized state in which she was unable to function at home or work. At the time that she was referred to me, I was working at the same private agency where she had earlier been a patient. During the 12 years in which she had previously been seen there, she had seen four different therapists, all of whom had left. When the fourth left, she refused to be reassigned. She did, however, agree to continue her antipsychotic medication through an outside psychiatrist, Dr. Z. This arrangement seemed to suffice until Wendy's mother died suddenly. Shortly thereafter, Dr. Z referred Wendy to me for weekly therapy.

Although Wendy is a few years older than I am, she has always greeted me in the waiting room with, "Hiiii, Miss Blotzer!" The effect made me feel as though she were a primary school student and I her teacher. Wendy's voice established distance and a hierarchy between us. And the hierarchy contained all her transference feelings toward authority figures—largely an amalgam of dependency and hostility. Her limitations were painful to her, and she realistically perceived most people as more capable and powerful than she. Because she lacked confidence in her own abilities and had deliberately shied away from experiences that would develop mastery, she viewed the world as populated by powerful others whom she needed to placate, please, cajole, or otherwise influence to do what she needed. She both needed them and resented her dependency on them. Furthermore, she wanted her needs to be met on *her* terms and was deeply suspicious of being controlled by others. Yet her experience had taught her that she must also placate and appease these powerful others lest she so anger them that they abandon her. She also feared her own anger. Her mental representations of these significant individuals are also shaky, and she fears that her anger could annihilate these images.

Such was the uneasy alliance that Wendy had reached with the world, and the alliance that she invited me to join. I would help her by doing what she asked, and she in turn would appease me by being a "good" patient. I wanted no part of it, and the first year of her therapy was a struggle as Wendy attempted to maneuver me into patronizing and controlling her, just as she tried to control me. This was her template for relationships, and a fundamental task of the therapy was to demonstrate a different way of relating, one based upon respect. Much of any therapy is based upon examining interactions. Transference, the patient's attempts to replicate important relationships with others in the here and now relationship with the therapist, forms much of the media for therapy. Yet during her first year in therapy, Wendy lacked the skills for examining her interactions. The burden fell heavily on me to maintain a therapeutic stance. I had to resist her attempts to maneuver me into patronizing her or getting angry at her.

I had to face it: Most individuals, myself included, found it hard to like Wendy. Almost everything about her evoked a negative reaction. As a therapist I knew that this was important material for therapy.

Although her physical appearance was slightly unusual due to the genetic syndrome that caused her mild mental retardation, she was not unattractive and, other than her voice, did not immediately strike one as being different. Rather, it was the way she related to others that created problems. Because she had almost no inner resources for tolerating the inevitable anxiety that came with waiting or being uncertain, she annoyed others with her constant questions and insistence upon having an immediate answer or resolution to any problem. So great was her inner terror that Wendy needed a world of rigid predictability. Much later in her therapy, she was able to talk about this and poignantly said, "I worried what would become of me."

There are both schizoid and autistic features to Wendy's manner of relating to others. She seems emotionally aloof from others and treats others almost as though they are things rather than persons. The rigid, limiting roles that she assigns to the important others in her life can make them feel like objects. At a time when I was concerned about Wendy's social isolation and was talking with her about arranging more social connections, Wendy could only tolerate this by saying that she needed a "driver" to take her places when she got bored. Relationships with Wendy must first begin on her own terms. Her terms require that the person first begin as someone who performs an important function for Wendy. Only after the person has met these functions and has been nonthreatening can Wendy consider a deeper relatedness. In this way Wendy controls the emotional intensity in her relationships, modulating it so that it is bearable to her. This rigidity with people is also her way of controlling the amount of novelty in her life.

It was only after I left the private nonprofit agency where I had seen Wendy for more than a year, and gave her the option of following me into my private practice, that Wendy and I were able to work on these issues on a deeper, more productive level. This shift in the depth of the therapy was not incidental. It reflected a level of commitment and stability that Wendy needed to feel in our relationship before she could safely face herself and her concerns. Wendy had been forced to change therapists four times before seeing me. Each of her previous therapists had left the agency, and, although each had worked diligently with Wendy to minimize the difficulties inherent in such changes, Wendy found each termination deeply unsettling. After the last therapist left, she refused to be reassigned and would only agree to meet bimonthly with a psychiatrist for medication monitoring. For three years this arrangement was sufficient, but then Wendy's mother died suddenly, and her father, who had a progressive neurological disease, moved to a nursing home. These events threatened to overwhelm Wendy's shaky equilibrium, and her psychiatrist, Dr. Z, urged her to begin weekly therapy with me. Wendy was deeply distrustful of this recommendation. At a time of great loss, she was uninterested in a reprise of the revolving door therapy that had characterized her previous experience at the agency. Reluctantly, she agreed with Dr. Z to consult with me about "practical matters."

For many reasons, Wendy was quite dubious about seeing me and wanted to rigidly circumscribe the relationship. She didn't want therapy if it meant talking about herself and her life. The thought of beginning a new relationship was more than she could tolerate in her overwhelmed state. She needed to block out external influences in order to hold on to her rapidly deteriorating sense of self. Getting involved with a new person felt too taxing on her already strained resources.

Perhaps because Wendy holds down a job, maintains her own apartment, and uses public transportation to get to work and therapy appointments, it is easy to overlook just how limited she is and the costs to her of this independence. Wendy manages these activities at considerable cost to her psychic energy. She copes by keeping the contours of her life very rigid and routinized. Indeed, she has very limited and rigid (not very effective) strategies for allowing newness into her life. Most commonly, she copes with her anxiety by saying no to new suggestions, as she did when Dr. Z suggested that she see me. When saying no proves impossible or when people continue to nudge her, she will accept their suggestion under narrow, rigidly circumscribed circumstances. What Wendy would admit was that she needed a "social worker for practical matters." Dr. Z was her psychiatrist for medication matters. On numerous occasions during our first weeks together, Wendy would repeat that I was her "social worker for practical matters." This was her way of managing her anxiety, of telling me not to ask too much of her, and of maintaining the distance that she needed in the relationship.

~

In this way Wendy began therapy. I was immediately struck by her rigidity, and the repetitiveness of her remarks. She felt very concrete and limited to me. I wondered whether she was capable of any meaningful examination of her life. At times during her early sessions I felt bored and trapped as I listened to her repetitive recitations delivered in a constricted fashion. Did she also feel bored and trapped? I believe that she did, but also that her boredom and constriction served powerful defensive functions. Her constriction was her way of keeping a psychic lid on the powerful, painful feelings that threatened to overwhelm her. Wendy's defenses are very primitive and limited. Lacking more flexible means for managing or modulating her intense feelings, she simply kept the lid on them as best she could. This defensive structure has kept her from deteriorating too badly, but it has come at an enormous price in energy and flexibility. As I look to the future with Wendy, I wonder to what extent she can develop greater flexibility once the acute distress in her life abates. As I write this, we are entering our third year together and she is demonstrating an expanded ability to cope more effectively.

Another reason that I felt frustrated and trapped as I sat with Wendy in those early months was because this was an unconscious communication from her. In order for her therapy to be successful, I had to experience something of the depths of her discomfort. If Wendy felt constricted and rigid in those early months, I felt hamstrung, as though I had little therapeutic leverage with which to help her. I knew that my ability to bear these feelings and to empathically stay connected to the stuck, shallow feeling was the key to helping her.

Wendy's parents, particularly her mother, had been her emotional lifeline. Although Wendy worked and had her own apartment, her life revolved around her mother. Her mother's death brought Wendy's world crashing down upon her. Although Wendy had a full-time job as an office clerk and her own apartment, she spent every weekend, holiday, snow day, sick day—any day that did not require her going to work—at her parents' house. Her apartment was more like a hotel. She ate breakfast and lunch at the cafeteria at work, and dinners in the dining hall of her apartment building. Wendy kept no food in her refrigerator and relied upon her mother to do her laundry and all of her shopping. Furthermore, she was in the habit of phoning her mother several times each day. The first thing she did when she got up in the morning was to telephone her mother. She'd next telephone her mother when she arrived at work, and at numerous times throughout the workday. At transitional times—whenever she felt bored, anxious, angry, sad—her habitual response was to lift the phone to talk with her mother. Wendy relied almost exclusively upon her mother to metabolize, regulate, and express her affects.

Wendy's inability to manage her own anxiety is perhaps her most debilitating deficit. Losing her mother meant not only that she lost the structure for a major portion of her life (the nonwork hours), it also meant that she lost the person who did most of her coping for her. Left without her mother, Wendy was left with no functional means for handling her anxiety, and this loss further intensified her anxiety.

Infant researchers and psychoanalysts have written about the process by which infants, with their primitive mental structures, manage intense emotions. Much as how, in utero, the mother filters toxins and passes nutrients through the umbilical cord, infants rely upon their mothers to contain and metabolize their intense feelings. Gradually, with good caregiving and the maturation of mental functions, the developing person learns to manage these states on her own. Wendy, however, had continued to rely upon her mother and had only the most primitive of her own abilities. Without mechanisms to soothe, distract, or otherwise distance herself from painful feelings, she experienced massive anxiety. She found waiting nearly unbearable, whether it was the waiting of not knowing or of waiting for me to return her call. And because she found waiting so unbearable, she would telephone incessantly or demand immediate, concrete answers to questions that had no immediate or concrete answers. This trait of hers was what others found so annoying. It was what our office staff, her work supervisor, and family friends responded to. The raw fashion in which she expressed her need for comfort tended to drive people away from her. It was easy to feel overburdened and overwhelmed by Wendy's demands. She could quickly deplete even the most vast reserves of patience and concern.

I found myself thinking very carefully about how to approach Wendy's therapy. She needed to mourn her losses, but without her parents available to provide emotional ballast, she could not safely manage her grief. Only when she developed stronger capacities for managing her feelings and felt herself to be less bereft could she begin the painful work of coming to terms with her mother's death and the impending death of her father. I realized that I needed to summon up all the patience and empathy that I could muster. Wendy and I would spend a long time in therapy, and much of that time would feel flat and repetitive. But rushing in too quickly would serve no purpose.

I did not challenge the terms that Wendy set for her therapy. During our first weeks together, I was struck by how rigid and concrete she seemed. At times I'd ask a question in an attempt to move her to a deeper level or to consider her emotional reactions. These attempts proved futile. Wendy seemed very organic to me, and I wondered whether our interactions would ever be different. I also realized that it was essential that I meet Wendy where she was. I had to find ways of unconsciously conveying empathy for her "stuckness." Hence, I decided to sit back and just focus upon listening to her and to deliberately not try to move her along. It was when I first did this that she began to soften, and she surprised me with flashes of insight or flexibility.

I've had this experience before with patients, and it's one of the first things that I try to get across when I supervise graduate students or clinicians who are new to working with persons who have intellectual disabilities. My sense is that we unconsciously convey our expectations: "Hurry up. Get with it. Let's do some real therapeutic work here." Our patients recoil from this, wanting to be taken on their own terms. Paradoxically, only when we as therapists let go of these expectations does the real work of therapy begin.

So it was with Wendy. After this settling-in period of a few weeks, during which she'd initially seemed very rigid and then demonstrated signs of softening, she began to focus intently upon her father. A new experimental drug was being tried for patients with his disorder. All of Wendy's anxiety seemed absorbed in wondering if the new drug would help her father. Would he get better and leave the nursing home? This was all that she could talk about for weeks. I wanted to deepen this line of inquiry, to mine it for all its therapeutic meaning and benefit. So I would ask Wendy what she thought would happen, what was her fantasy, how she envisioned her life in either scenario. I wanted to at least draw out the theme, if not to develop variations on it. Wendy would have none of this. She stubbornly, rigidly, and perseveratively played the same notes with an aching lack of artistry, "Can the drug help my father?"

One day she then and there demanded that I phone her father's nursing home to ask about the drug. I resisted and tried to draw out her reasons for the urgent request. Not knowing what was wrapped up in her request of me, I was hesitant to comply until I better understood it. Yet as I sought more details from Wendy, she became increasingly agitated, demanding, and hostile. I felt almost bullied by her. Wendy was making the issue into a power struggle as I simply delayed until I better understood her motivation. Finally, Wendy told me that Pastor R, the family friend who took her to see her father, had forbidden her to contact the nursing home. It seemed that she had gone through a period of "pestering" the nursing home staff with persistent telephone calls. To control this, Pastor R had forbidden her to call again and said that he would be the conduit for all communication. This was a classic example of Wendy's difficulties with authority, and this transference was triggered when I did not immediately accede to Wendy's request to call the nursing home. Wendy bitterly resented her pastor's rule, but was terrified to break it lest she so anger him that he refuse to ever again take her to visit her father.

I decided to be very forthright with Wendy. I told her that I disagreed with her pastor. I told her that I thought she had a right to telephone the nursing home and that I would personally telephone Pastor R to tell him so. I reassured her that I would emphatically support her need and right to contact her father's physicians. "You're his daughter," I said. "It's your job to see that he gets all the help that he needs. You have a right to talk to them." I think that Wendy felt respected by my validation of her filial role. I really was unwilling to tolerate her being cast aside, and she knew this.

Equally directly, I told Wendy that her repetitive telephone calls and pestering demands drove people away and made them not want to help her. I felt tactless, but I think that Wendy needed me to be direct and to confront her. It is also possible that what feels like tactless directness is actually essential for helping Wendy understand interpersonal issues. I suspect that she lacks the ability to read more subtle social cues. For example, most of us when we stop to chat with a neighbor can read the signals—the brief answers, the looking around or at a watch, the closed body language—that conveys the message, "Leave me alone." But many individuals are less proficient at this decoding of social signals. They are the ones who don't seem to get our subtle cues. They are the dinner guests who show no signs of leaving despite audible and frequent yawns from the host. We feel annoyed and irritated with these individuals. They either force us to be more direct than we want to be, or, if we are uncomfortable being so direct, to tolerate their intrusions while we simmer with resentment. I suspect that difficulty reading more subtle social cues accounts for a significant portion of Wendy's difficulties with others.

This session seemed to mark a turning point in our relationship. I think on that day she realized what was unique about our therapeutic relationship—that I would talk to her about her behavior while remaining connected to her, that I would not enter into power struggles with her, and that I was not interested in replaying the hostile–dependent relationship that was her template. These latter interactions were emblematic of all her frustrations with the more powerful others who populated her world.

~

Wendy's style is to repetitively focus upon an issue or theme for what feels to me like an endless amount of time. But I have learned patience and found that Wendy's pace is the right one for her. It clearly is the process by which Wendy works through her concerns. And she does this best when I interfere the least. On occasion Wendy has sensed my restlessness with her pace. Wendy had been talking for some months about how hard it was for her to make the sudden adjustment to staying all the time at her apartment: "Other people leave home when their parents are still alive. I wish I'd gotten on my own sooner." I was listening with what I thought was patience throughout this exchange when Wendy said, "Pastor R said I should look on the bright side," while scanning my face for a reaction to this suggestion. I wondered if she had sensed some impatience from me and had obliged by suggesting an alternative. I replied, "It can be hard to look on the bright side when you are feeling so sad." Wendy paused and looked long at me. I think that she was used to people shutting her off. Her way of asking if I was going to shut her off was to say, "Pastor R said I should look on the bright side," and to see if I agreed. Initially, I felt solid about suggesting the possibility that Wendy needed to do something other than look on the bright side. Although I believe that it was true that my response showed respect for both the depth of her feeling and for her autonomy, I believe that it missed the other part of her request. To some extent Wendy was asking me to help regulate her affect, much as her mother had done. This notion was supported by material in subsequent sessions.

For several weeks Wendy had been interjecting, "Know what I mean?" as she talked to me about how difficult the changes precipitated by her mother's death had been. Initially, I hadn't really noticed or thought about this comment, viewing it more as conversational static or background noise. But for some reason, perhaps because she intensified it, her "Know what I mean?" at the end of sentences filtered up to that place in my consciousness where I reflect more deeply upon the meaning of statements from my patients. I asked Wendy about it, and her response made it clear that she genuinely wanted to know if I knew what she was going through. She was searching for something more from me. She didn't feel that I truly understood or empathized with her. I tried asking her what she needed me to do in order for her to feel empathized with, but she was unable to make use of this question.

Later, I consulted with Dr. Z about this. Dr. Z had seen both Wendy and her mother together and described Wendy's mother as a sociable, talkative person who did the emoting for both of them. Wendy questioned whether I understood her because I didn't overtly express her emotionality. Instead, I created a space for Wendy to express whatever was within her. But the flip side of this was that Wendy felt lonely. She'd had little experience at being a separate person. Instead she had been merged with her mother, who expressed the affect for both of them. Being with me—and the quiet, unintrusive space that I provided—left her feeling alone and not understood.

Staying empathically connected to Wendy was at times difficult for me. It took more conscious mental effort on my part. Try as I might to listen patiently to Wendy, something else intervened. Being with her felt awkward at times. She taxed my energy and patience in many ways. At times I felt bored and restless. Throughout the process, my observing ego would note this and I could continue to work at staying connected to her. There are times when our work still feels tedious, and I often have to remind myself of what Wendy might be feeling. Part of the exhaustion and tedium is due to the constricted and repetitive quality of Wendy's speech. There's a strong stimulus-bound quality to her. She can only deal with a small piece of her experience at a time, and she talks about this in a very restricted fashion. There's little elaboration and embellishment. The monotone that she speaks in combines with her lack of emotional expressiveness to choke off all feeling. At times Wendy will be talking about issues that clearly cause her great sadness, and I will have to remind myself of her sadness because she does not show it. This is the other aspect of Wendy's that makes it so difficult for her to have friends. Even when she is hurting deeply, she seldom evokes tender feelings from others. Her emotional constriction and general rigidity not only keep her own feelings at safe distance; these same factors keep others at safe distance. Wendy is a woman both alone and lonely.

What sustains me in my work with her is the deep conviction that the tedium that I sometimes feel is not all that there is. Certainly, one reason I feel that tedium is because Wendy is projecting her intolerable sense of emptiness into me, along with her terror at that emptiness. So my challenge as her therapist is to accept her pace and to pay careful attention to the reactions that she evokes in me. Wendy continues to amaze me. Just when I think that she is hopelessly perseverating, she will demonstrate genuine insight or flexibility.

After a year in therapy, Wendy seemed more able to examine her life and feelings. Several factors accounted for this. Perhaps most importantly, I had offered her the option of following me into my private practice when I left the agency where we'd begun our work together. Wendy was quick to accept this offer and surprised me by readily stating her reason, "I've had enough change." She then went on to list the various therapists whom she'd seen over her career as a patient and said, "I want to stay with you, if that's all right." My move and offer to continue with Wendy gave her a sense of stability, and she sensed my commitment to her. The passage of time and experience had also helped Wendy. Although still rigid and emotionally constricted, she showed greater flexibility and a greater capacity for reflection than I would have thought possible, given her earlier presentation. Recently, when talking about how her pastor had encouraged her to spend more time apart from her parents, she said, "Pastor R saw it coming. I didn't."

Regret was a prominent theme with Wendy for many months during this second year of therapy. She regretted not having become more gradually independent of her parents. She talked about how others had urged her to spend some weekends apart from her parents while they were both still well, but she had not wanted to. Part of the problem for Wendy is her very limited ability to anticipate consequences. She lacks adequate imaginative capacity to project herself into the abstract future. She never really believed that her parents would die. Unfortunately for Wendy, the significant others in her life see the likely outcome long before she does. When they try to encourage her to anticipate the outcome, she feels that they are trying to control or boss her. On some level Wendy knows that she is less able than others to anticipate and plan ahead. Her focus upon her regret was her way of expressing this. The larger conflict created by the intersection of Wendy's inner conflict about her limited anticipatory ability has combined with her conflicts about dependency to make it even harder for her to use the ability that she does have and to accept assistance from others. I see this issue as an important focus of our therapy and look for openings to address it.

During this time when Wendy was talking about wishing she'd done things differently, Wendy's supervisor experienced a death in her family. Wendy has a very complicated relationship with her supervisor, Caroline, and I periodically talk by phone with the two of them together. "Caroline's sad, too," said Wendy. "Her mother died. But it's not like she lost her home. I lost my home. Caroline has her own home." Wendy was comparing her loss to Caroline's loss. What she said next surprised me. "Caroline's father must hurt the most. He had children by her." Wendy was rank-ordering the intensity of these losses, based upon the closeness of the relationship. Wendy compared her grief to that of "a college graduate" losing her parents, and felt that to lose the person by whom one had had children was a deeper loss than her own loss (as an adult) of her parents. Never before had Wendy shown such insight into others, nor demonstrated the ability to step back and reflect upon how her experience compared with that of others.

~

During this second year the reality of Wendy's losses sank in more deeply, and she began adjusting to her changed circumstances. A concrete example of these changed circumstances was the preparations to sell the family home. Again, Wendy's pastor was her guide in this process. Pastor R gave her plenty of lead time to adjust to the idea.

For many months Wendy and I had been discussing the loss of the family home, and Wendy was coming to terms with it. "It's not like I can live there. It's too far from work. Pastor R said it's better to have a family live there." Wendy began one session by telling me that there had just been a yard sale to clear out the house. She was able to say that this had been "hard" and "sad" for her, but then moved on to other topics once this pain had been acknowledged.

Interestingly, this was the first time that Wendy had talked about feeling sad. I believe this indicated that for the first time she felt safe enough to admit this feeling into awareness. About 4 months prior to this, I had jumped the gun. Wendy had taken a week's vacation from work and spent the entire time in her apartment. With few social contacts in her building and with few internal resources for managing her free time, Wendy was left alone with her grief without the distractions or social support of her job. When she came to therapy the next week and told me about it, I sensed that it had been a pretty awful week for her. When I suggested that she might have felt sad and lonely, Wendy adamantly corrected me. The only feeling that she would admit to was being bored. I accepted this, and we would periodically revisit "being bored" in the ensuing months. For Wendy, a person who is out of touch with and frightened by strong feelings, "bored" is the dysphoric affect that she can safely acknowledge. Wendy and I were actually able to do quite a bit of productive therapy around the notion of "being bored." Talking about this was a bridge to allowing herself to admit that she did want more contact with others, and to considering broadening the narrow confines of her life. I think that our work with "bored" allowed her to safely move to "sad."

~

Wendy's anxiety has significantly lessened, and she does seem to be managing it more on her own. One reason for her lessened anxiety is that she now has more "answers." Wendy finds uncertainty extremely difficult to tolerate. This is due to a number of factors—her limited ability to anticipate and to plan ahead, her limited strategies for soothing herself or otherwise managing her anxiety, and her terror at being unable to manage new situations. Early in her therapy she was nearly beside herself with worry, wondering whether a new experimental drug would help her father. It consumed her. So intense was her focus on this issue that her work supervisor phoned me to complain that Wendy was totally ineffective at work and was spending all her work hours phoning the pharmacy and the nursing home to ask about experimental drugs for her father.

Because I sensed that the anxiety of uncertainty was intolerable for Wendy, and that she needed a concrete answer to this question in order to move on, she and I arranged to talk together by telephone with her father's physician. Beforehand, we made a list of questions that she wanted to ask. Her father's physician was completely frank and said that Wendy's father was too advanced in his condition to benefit from any experimental drugs. He outlined a grim prognosis. As painful as this news was for Wendy, she coped much more effectively once she knew what to expect. The prior uncertainty had been intolerable to her.

Recently Wendy wondered whether her father would always recognize her. Sensing that she knew that he would not, I replied that he would probably lose the ability to recognize others. With Wendy I am much more definite and unambiguous in my statements. She would have been ill-served if I'd responded to her inquiry by asking what she thought. Once I acknowledged his inevitable deterioration, Wendy was able to talk more about what this meant for her. For the first time she acknowledged that she did not know what to do with her father when they visited. Concretely, I told her that she could hold his hand and say, "Dad, this is Wendy, your daughter," and that she could simply talk about what she'd been doing. She seemed relieved when I told her that her father could no longer converse, but that she could do the talking for both of them. This sort of practical, concrete advice often serves as a bridge to enable Wendy to share more of her concerns. To attempt to draw her out before doing this is counterproductive. My approach to Wendy illustrates the oscillation between dynamic and supportive approaches. Our work together is oriented toward transformative work, but with Wendy such transformation is achieved by first strengthening her ego functioning.

The validity of this approach is being increasingly reinforced by the growing insight and flexibility that Wendy demonstrates. A recent session shows her ability to examine interactions, to admit into awareness and to express a greater range of emotion, and to actively explain herself.

~

Wendy began the session by asking about her father's prognosis. I suggested that perhaps it might be time for us to schedule another phone consultation with his doctor. Eager to do this, and continuing to have difficulties waiting, she asked how soon I could arrange this. I replied that if the doctor was available we could probably talk with him during our regularly scheduled session the next week. After having me repeat and clarify this a few times, Wendy next said, "It's settled. You'll call. I won't bug you anymore." I was surprised by this comment. It reflected her growing ability to examine herself as well as being a reference to the time when she had relentlessly demanded that I phone the nursing home. We were able to talk about the earlier occasion as well as the current situation and how her response now was so much different. "I got a grip on myself," said Wendy.

When I mentioned how hard it must be for her to tolerate the uncertainty of her father's condition, not knowing how long he'll live nor the pace of his deterioration, she replied, "That's why I bugged Dr. S more. He said he didn't know. I needed to know." She went on to tell me that while her mother was still alive that she (Wendy) had repetitively called her father's doctor because he was unable to give her a definitive prognosis. "That made it worse because he didn't know. I was afraid of what would become of us," said Wendy, explaining how the doctor's uncertainty had only made her more frantic. This depth of insight, explaining that she would call persistently because of the uncertainty, was something that I had not seen before from her. In some ways her "bugging" others represented a nearly manic defense against sadness. She then went on to talk about how she felt when, in response to her too frequent calls, Pastor R had forbidden her to phone the new doctor. "I was robbed of talking to his doctor sooner. I brought it on myself. It's half my fault." We then moved on to discussing the outcome of this conversation with the new doctor—being told that her father was too advanced to benefit from the new drug. As her eyes welled with tears, she said, "I'm disappointed it (the drug) didn't work. Real disappointed." We began for the first time to talk in depth about how hard it is for her to manage her anxiety, and that she doesn't mean to "bug" people, but simply does so because she doesn't know what else to do with her worried feelings. This session, with her insight and greater expression of feeling and her ability to examine her reactions and interaction, stands in stark contrast to her earlier constriction.

~

Because Wendy does not have family available to her I feel an extra level of responsibility and find myself concerned with the practical aspects of her life. I worry about her health. She's had some disturbing physical symptoms, and I'm not always confident that she accurately reports these to her doctor. I worry about her isolation and about her future. Pastor R and his wife have provided untold practical assistance to her. They regularly take her to visit her father—a round-trip for them of nearly 100 miles. They took her to get new glasses and also to buy new clothes for her. It was they who discovered that her apartment was filthy and arranged for homemaker services. I want to ensure that Wendy has an alternate way of getting such practical assistance in the event that Pastor and Mrs. R are no longer able to help. Only recently has Wendy been able to consider alternatives and allow more services into her life. Her reluctance stems both from her habitual reluctance to try anything new as well as her fear that she would see Pastor R less if he didn't have a practical reason for being in her life. Wendy likes her pastor, as much for himself as for the linkage he provides to her earlier life with her parents.

~

In addition to concerning myself with practical matters, I also find myself in periodic contact with the other significant persons in Wendy's life—Pastor R and Caroline, Wendy's work supervisor. So that Wendy does not feel talked about behind her back, in addition to a signed authorization release from Wendy, I require that Pastor R and Caroline first tell Wendy if they are planning to call me. Similarly, I always ask Wendy first if I want to call Pastor R or Caroline, and I review with her what I want to discuss with them. This collaboration, although unusual with most adult patients, is necessary because of Wendy's vulnerability and because she can also be very difficult. On numerous occasions, Caroline has phoned me at her wit's end, ready to take adverse job action against Wendy. Wendy's job is an important organizing factor in her life, and the consequences for her would be devastating if she lost it. She finds it very difficult to cope with unstructured time, such as weekends and vacations. Her job gives her life structure and keeps her from becoming too isolated.

Because my contact with Caroline departs from the traditional notions about contact with others, I have carefully evaluated whether it is appropriate. I have considered whether I am involved because no one else is available to do so, or because this role requires my skills as a therapist and my relationship as Wendy's therapist. In Wendy's case I am motivated by exigencies of the situation and the need for a clinical approach in addressing her work problems.

Although Wendy has now held the same job for more than 10 years, it has not been problem-free. Wendy's length of stay is more a testament to her supervisor's tolerance and less a reflection of good performance. At times Wendy's job performance has been wholly inadequate. Caroline has complained that Wendy rushes through tasks, completing them in a sloppy fashion. On occasion Wendy has refused to do the tasks assigned to her, and she and Caroline have gotten into power struggles. Despite it all, Caroline feels sorry for Wendy and allows her to get away with things that would cost other employees their jobs. But periodically Wendy will do something that exhausts the limits of Caroline's tolerance, and Caroline will phone me.

Wendy's interaction with Caroline is problematic. Wendy can be extremely trying, and Caroline has received no training on how to supervise employees with intellectual deficits. Furthermore, Wendy's style of relating typically evokes annoyance rather than tenderness. Recently, Caroline told me that she'd "caught" Wendy crying at work and responded by asking Wendy if she was having "a pity party for herself." Although I was stunned by the callousness of Caroline's response, I could understand the source of the callousness. Caroline is not an insensitive person, but Wendy can frustrate and annoy even the most saintly person. The cumulative effect of Wendy's defensive structure, largely organized to keep her own feelings at a safe distance, also functions to keep others at distance. Wendy's presentation makes it hard to both feel and relate to her pain. Intellectually, Caroline can remind herself of Wendy's need for tenderness, but Wendy seldom evokes tender feelings.

Because of these complexities and the capacity for their relationship to become sadistic, I asked Caroline and Wendy to phone me together on a regular basis so that we can discuss how work is going. My goal in doing so is to provide Wendy with regular feedback from Caroline and to give Caroline practice at talking over concerns directly with Wendy, rather than running directly to me. These regular phone conferences also give me a broader perspective on Wendy's difficulties and on how she is coping. Wendy's performance has been improving since we began this process.

Talking with Caroline has also provided important glimpses into the social ecology of Wendy's worksite. Wendy's co-workers frequently complain about her to Caroline. Wendy's social skills are problematic. Although she has many skills, these are not firmly established, and they desert her in times of stress. She evokes and provokes negative reactions from many of her co-workers. Reportedly, she interrupts them constantly and does not respond to subtle social cues—the clipped answers, the restless body language that telegraph, "Leave me alone. I'm busy." But rather than deal directly with her, they complain to Caroline, expecting her to "fix" Wendy. So overburdened did Caroline feel that she told me, "I'm tired of being Wendy's wet nurse." The imagery is not accidental. So unfiltered and unmodulated are Wendy's needs at times, that people fear being used up. One of my goals has been to extricate Caroline from this position.

Wendy's co-workers reflect the larger culture's discomfort with disability. They alternate between infantilizing and pitying her when they project their own vulnerabilities onto her, and between hating and rejecting her when she expresses the socially inept, needy, demanding, stupid parts of themselves. Because they find it hard to tolerate their own ambivalence, they act in ways that make Caroline feel solely responsible for Wendy. But again, because of their ambivalence, they criticize Caroline for being "mean" when she loses patience with Wendy. As the repository for the projections and conflicts of Wendy's co-workers, Caroline finds herself feeling resentful yet discomfitted at having such feelings. Predictably, her interactions with Wendy alternated between an overly lenient tolerance and anger at being her "wet nurse."

My goal has been to assist Caroline in removing herself from this untenable situation so that she could have a more constructive relationship with Wendy. I did so by acknowledging the legitimacy of her mixed feelings. People who deal with Wendy often feel bad about their negative reactions to her. And feeling bad about their response binds them up, preventing them from relating to her more authentically, which is ultimately more productive. This thick soup of conflicted feelings and defenses against these feelings must be penetrated before real relationships are possible.

My first step with Caroline was to openly acknowledge how difficult Wendy can be and that she does both evoke and provoke negative reactions. This seemed to detoxify her feelings and enabled her to move from defending against these feelings to thinking productively about how she wanted to respond to Wendy. Their relationship is steadily shifting, with Caroline feeling freed to be a supervisor who can set appropriate standards and hold Wendy accountable. With their relationship less a muddy mix of transference phenomenon, and with clear standards and feedback, Wendy's performance has been improving. Wendy is pleased to have a more adult relationship with Caroline and recently told me how she handled what previously would have been a problematic issue between them. Caroline had been telling Wendy that she hadn't been doing one of her tasks adequately. Wendy found herself becoming defensive but caught herself. Relating the story to me she said, "To cool down, I asked her how I was doing."

~

Finally, Wendy's case raises questions about consent. Wendy has a history of psychotic breakdowns. Wendy's attitude toward her psychotic illness is noteworthy. She simply denies that it exists and does not talk about it. On several occasions since her first breakdown, Wendy has insisted that the psychiatrist treating her wean her off of all medications. On each occasion, the outcome has been disastrous, with Wendy rapidly deteriorating into psychotic, disorganized thinking, becoming nonfunctional at work and home, and ending up in the psychiatric ward. Dr. Z, who has twice seen Wendy decompensate when off medication, now has an agreement with Wendy that they will only reconsider medication at 6-month intervals. This structures the issue and makes it less of a power struggle.

When dealing with patients who have intellectual limits, consent issues can become more complicated, and therapists sometimes assume expanded roles. Both Dr. Z and I feel more responsible for Wendy because she has no family to help her and because her deficient judgment concerns us. There are times when I will suggest something to Wendy that I think will be helpful—perhaps homemaker services or other drop-in assistance. Because Wendy becomes highly anxious when anything new is suggested and habitually says no, I do not accept her initial refusal as the final word on the subject. Recognizing her intense need to remain in control and her resentment of intrusions, I never argue the point with her. Rather, I plant the seed for her to think about, and I reaffirm that the decision is hers. But I clearly do seek to guide her more than I would another patient. I think carefully about this and regularly consult with colleagues for their views on the issue; however, I believe that my intensified role is appropriate, given Wendy's needs and limits.

I strongly support Dr. Z's approach to Wendy's medication. We run great risks when we think we know better than our patients. We risk violating their rights and dignity and risk abusing our professional responsibilities. Yet I believe that we must also recognize when a patient's judgment is impaired. After all, does the "no" from the patient who habitually says "no" truly constitute informed consent? Although the potential for abuse is great, I believe we must be willing to consider these issues, and to tolerate the inevitable tensions that arise from trying to balance these concerns.

~

A number of issues stand out as I review Wendy's therapy. Perhaps most striking is the impact anxiety places on her organic presentation. When overcome by massive anxiety, Wendy functions at a more limited level and is much less flexible. What appears to be an organically based deficit can actually be a defensive adaptation. Those of us who treat persons with intellectual disabilities must be constantly working to distinguish these defensive functions from the true intellectual limits of our patients. As I look to the future with Wendy, a major goal is to help her manage her anxiety in ways that give her greater flexibility.

I also feel the need to reiterate how important it was for me to meet her on her own terms. Although the currency of the phrase "start where the client is" has become devalued from overuse, it was absolutely essential to the therapy that I accepted her "stuckness" and did not press her to go further than she was able to at that point. In the case of Wendy, where she started from is quite removed from where she is now.

Wendy's initial interactions with me, which typified her difficulties with the powerful others who populate her life, show signs of change, both intrapsychically and in the external world. We've had no reprise of the earlier power struggles, and not only is she learning that our relationship can be different, but she is also relating in more adult ways to Pastor R and to Caroline.

The power of empathy never ceases to amaze me in my clinical work. Once Wendy's experience has been empathically acknowledged, she can move forward to reflect upon it. It's as though my empathy is the catalyst that allows her observing ego to function.

I'm also reminded of how challenging it can be to work with the Wendys of the world. It took me some time to understand her well enough to work effectively with her. I now feel quite fond of her, but there are still occasions that challenge me to look past her immediate presentation. Only by paying careful attention to what she evokes in me can we remain appropriately connected. Perhaps this is why, with patients like Wendy, it is so essential to work with the important others in their lives. Caroline and Pastor R both want to be helpful to her. By acknowledging to them that indeed Wendy can be trying, they are able to bring their own observing egos to their interactions with Wendy and respond in ways that are helpful, rather than hurtful.

Last, I am struck by how different she seems to me. From our first interaction, I knew that she would invite me to patronize her and that I would have to work hard to maintain a therapeutic stance. I sensed that there was more to her, but I am truly startled by her insight and depth as she has emerged from behind her mask. As I write this, I have been seeing Wendy for years and will probably see her indefinitely. In many ways she has improved dramatically. I remain optimistic about how much farther she can go.

6

R.J.

Long-Term Therapy with a Disagreeable Man

Richard Ruth

There is a pervasive fantasy among theorists, advocates, health care providers, and even among people with disabilities that disabilities are discrete entities that come singly. In fact, much historic thinking in the disability rights movement was formulated around a paradigm of a male paraplegic with no compounding difficulties. His health—these fantasies are prototypically about men; for reasons that cannot possibly be incidental, they begin falling apart when you try to extend them to women—is robust and stable; he is brighter than average, with deep wellsprings of drive and perseverance; and he is psychologically mature and well adjusted, probably because of the many fine qualities with which his purification in the crucible of disability has endowed him. If the society would only build more ramps and better bathrooms, he would be fine.

This fantasy comes from a good place. It embodies the powerful collective reaction of people with disabilities, given voice through our civil rights movement, against a dominant medical, mental health, and rehabilitation establishment that focuses on our deficits, denies our strengths and gifts, tells us what we cannot do, and then works to make its pessimistic predictions a reality.

We are right to reject these limitations. Since the founding of the independent living movement in the 1970s, people with disabilities have been working to create totally new ideas and models of what we can do and who we can be. We have done good work thus far.

Still, there is this fantasy of the single disability (using the term fantasy here in its clinical sense) and the tendency to oversimplify the needs of people with disabilities. Many people with disabilities do *not* fit the model of an otherwise perfect paraplegic. And there are reasons why this is so: Often the devastation done by chronic illness and/or disability is more pervasive; or the vulnerabilities, somatic and psychological, caused by one disability make for the acquisition of others. We fall, get into accidents, or are chronically stressed out and get sick when our resistance is low; and we may not recover as quickly as persons without disabilities, or without lingering wounds. Some of the vulnerabilities are economic—we can't afford health care, medicines, adequate technology, or food; some are social—we are targets of oppression, assault, and neglect. Doctors often refuse to understand us, and do thoughtless or damaging things. Thus, the model person with disabilities, if there is such a thing, may have multiple physical disabilities and accompanying cognitive and emotional issues.

Part of the story of the disability rights and independent living movements is that organizations created for the mutual radical empowerment of persons with discrete and delimited disabilities soon found themselves flooded with persons with severe and multiple disabilities, with much cognitive, emotional, and communicational involvement. Traditional service systems have often been very glad to pass off these people to alternative or innovative systems—less out of a desire to try creative possibilities than to get rid of problem "cases." The best and strongest parts of the disability movement (both organizations like ADAPT and individual therapists) have worked with these involved persons.

~

My work with R.J. illustrates the difficulties involved with someone with multiple physical and mental disabilities. R.J. came to me through his attorney. I took the case seriously when this remarkably tolerant and competent lawyer told me R.J. was one of the most difficult persons with whom he had ever worked. He was rude, prone to temper outbursts, not very bright, demanding, narcissistic, self-sabotaging, outrageous, and frequently in crises, during which he would haughtily demand resolutions from others. He was gay and made thoughtless and sometimes dangerous choices about partners who bruised and abused him. The lawyer was representing him in a personal injury suit, stemming from an incident in which he had been hit by a bus and left with a bad knee and leg. This case was drawn out and complicated. R.J. was unable to work and had no source of income, and, as the case was dragging on interminably, he was becoming increasingly desperate and impoverished. He would come to the lawyer with awful mixtures of intense, unfiltered need and rage. For 2 years the attorney had been trying to get him to see a therapist, but he had angrily refused. He claimed he wasn't crazy; he had been hit by a bus, and he needed money and relief from pain, not words. Recently, he'd been feeling so bad that he finally decided to seek therapy, but only if the lawyer could guarantee that the therapist was pro-gay and very good.

Once the lawyer told me all this, he quickly became apologetic and doubtful. He liked me; he was not sure about saddling me with this. Could I take it? And did I think I could help R.J.? I had my own doubts, considering the challenge and the probable delays in compensation.

~

R.J., when I first met him, was in his early 40s, an unassuming-looking man whose somewhat childlike face would at moments grimace with pain. His right leg would not straighten, and he walked somewhat tentatively and with a limp. He was slightly overweight. A small scar was visible in the center of his forehead, and he wore outdated clothing. R.J.'s first session was full of crises and challenges, which he described in a narrative full of mispronounced words and sparse vocabulary, lacking in coherent organization and chronology. He seemed mentally retarded, and I wondered whether the attorney had not known this or just had not told me. There was also a perseverative quality to R.J.'s thinking, and he demonstrated serious emotional lability, which immediately made me suspect brain damage.

R.J. told me he was diabetic and had no money for needles, testing strips, or an adequate diet. He lived with an older man who took his money, treated him like a servant, and berated him all the time. But he did not want to leave him and was afraid he would be kicked out now that he was no longer bringing home an income. He had been a food-service worker before his accident, but he had been suspended from work, as a safety risk, because of his disability, and was unsure whether he would be allowed to take up a different position or be discharged. Nor was he sure he could still do this job, although part of him wanted to.

I listened with attention and as much empathy as I could muster. As R.J.'s barrage of complaints chipped quickly away at the reserves of empathy in my heart, I felt my facial muscles becoming more and more rigid—the mask of a therapist about to shut off the client's words.

And it *was* a barrage. R.J. gave me no space to respond to any of his urgent crises, or to say much of anything. My every pause and hesitation was a crime, my every hint of uncertainty an attack on his credibility and on the legitimacy of his disability. But he realized two thirds of the way through the first hour that he was being hard on me. He was sure—because the lawyer told him so, not I thought because he had noticed my confused, wounded, wholehearted suffering through the last half-hour—that I would do everything I could to help him. He then listed a series of requests for advocacy and concrete assistance. We drifted farther by the minute from the tranquil shores of psychoanalysis. My response was irrelevant. The work had begun.

My summer vacation was to begin 2 weeks later. With another patient, I might have postponed beginning therapy until I returned. In R.J.'s case, given the intensity of his needs, I felt compelled to begin immediately. I briefly wondered where the boundary lay between objective needs and the feelings R.J. was evoking in me, but I plunged ahead. I paid a price for this, however. The evening I landed at my destination, 3,000 miles away, my answering service reached me with an emergency call. R.J. was being evicted by his lover; he had no money, nowhere to go, no one else to turn to. I listened, feeling impotent, enraged, confused, and in pain, conscious that something was being projected into me and that my job was to contain, metabolize, and honor the urgency of the crisis by coming up with some response that worked. After 20 minutes, I succeeded in helping R.J. to realize that, even though he felt the edict was unloving and unfair, he had little to gain by trying to salvage the relationship and little chance of persuading the roommate to change his decision. Though other feelings were present, the two men hated each other. We also established that the eviction would not take effect for 3 weeks and that there was time to meet and strategize after I returned. The practical advice I offered was important; however, even more important was that R.J. had projected into me an accurate sense of how he felt, and I hadn't counterattacked or left the field.

Soon after my return from vacation, I asked R.J. if he would let me do some psychological testing with him. Although I don't often request such testing, I felt I needed to know at the outset some things about his cognitive level, the depth and dynamics of his emotional disturbance, his personality style, and whether he had an acquired brain injury. I considered referring him to a colleague for testing, but I was not sure R.J. would allow another therapeutic figure into his life, having so long resisted coming to me. Even if he consented to seeing a colleague, the splitting might be overwhelming and the transference might shatter beyond hope of repair. Further, I was pessimistic that I could identify a competent colleague willing to take on such a complex diagnostic assessment of this disagreeable character and with such a remote prospect of reimbursement. When I broached the possibility of testing to him, R.J.'s reactions suggested that he liked the notion, for narcissistic reasons, of having an extra dose of undivided attention; in addition, he unconsciously heard my request as a willingness to think about him seriously and in depth. He experienced the request as a secure holding, and that seemed a good and safe reason for proceeding.

R.J.'s IQ scores were in the borderline average range for verbal functions and in the low end of the low average range for nonverbal functions. He was not retarded, but he had significant receptive, expressive, and process dysphasia. In no cognitive subdomain did his functioning rise to the average range. Educational testing showed he was functionally illiterate. He had a modest store of sight words, could sound out words and spell at a second-grade level, and knew basic math facts but quickly got flustered and made mistakes with multidigit arithmetic problems. He did not know fractions, percentages, or simple word problems. This was a profile suggesting serious, multifaceted learning disabilities, almost certainly predating the accident. His attention and concentration were very poor, patchily established, and easily shattered by mild environmental distractors.

A neuropsychological battery made it clear that a brain injury had occurred with the accident, compounding his problems and primarily affecting emotional regulation and the so-called executive functions, organized in the frontal lobes. Abilities to integrate, smooth, plan, and reason were affected. Almost no abstract reasoning capacity was preserved. Motor planning and fluency were compromised. Balance was shaky, and proprioception—the capacity to instinctively know where body parts are in space—was not good.

Testing of emotional status and personality indicated that before his accident R.J. had internalized messages that he was worthless and bad from very early in his development. He lacked feelings of secure attachment. Hunger for nurturance was long unmet and festering. His core experiences were organized in a paranoid-schizoid mode. The template of his defenses, in symbolic terms, was like that of an infant, sadistically attacking a breast experienced as ungiving and inadequate; because this was never ultimately gratifying, it evoked feelings of deep shame so strong it challenged basic ideas R.J. had about himself, he unconsciously neutralized his sadistic wishes by internalizing a belief that he was incompetent and impotent. Beyond this, there was significant test evidence of an element of biologically based, endogenous depression.

R.J.'s accidental injury had resonated against this base. It restimulated the full measure of his frustrated hungers, rage against primary objects (i.e., internal "parents"), feelings of helplessness and despair, paranoid suspiciousness, and aggressive sadism. He had internalized a sense that the accident had somehow legitimized his limitations and therefore stopped trying. R.J. released into the external world the toxic psychological "waste products"—the accident's validation of his most pessimistic beliefs and extensive narcissistic wounds. When he perceived others as having symbolically taken up these ideas and feelings he had tried to get rid of—as, for instance, when his lover disavowed him, or when I asked him a question and he forgot it, before remembering he couldn't answer it—he would attack others savagely. This produced conflict, between pleasure in the fleeting experience of agency and power and feeling flooded by a momentary awareness of how unfair and primal this all was.

Clearly, R.J. was in severe, chronic pain. There were moments when he was remarkably undefended, and the expression of his physical distress was hauntingly unadorned and direct.

~

R.J. was from a small town with few resources in a nearby state, whose young people either relocated, never to return, or were consigned to narrow and limited lives. His working-class parents were harsh, prejudice-ridden, stingy with their attention, and rigid and hypercritical in their beliefs. They dealt with their own deep unhappiness either by turning inward or by direct discharge, through aggression or drinking. They passed on this coping strategy to their children, so that R.J., the youngest of five, was the butt of his older siblings' derision and harassment.

R.J. attended special education classes for students with learning disabilities until he dropped out after the eighth grade. He doesn't recall much about his school years, except that he didn't learn much and never felt his teachers cared much about him or expected much from him. Not until the fourth year of therapy did I learn that R.J.'s brother began sexually molesting him shortly before he left school; this abuse continued regularly for 4 years thereafter. This is still much too painful and complex a topic for R.J. to discuss openly with me. For now, he seems relieved that I am aware of the abuse and that perhaps I can keep it in mind as I work with him.

R.J. did unskilled work for a few years. He married as a teenager, hoping he could escape his parents' harshness and become heterosexual at the same time. He fathered a son and shortly thereafter had a depressive breakdown, which in the long run was probably lifesaving.

R.J.'s wife divorced him in the course of his several-months' hospitalization, during which adult-onset diabetes was also diagnosed.

After the worst of the depression was over, he went to a halfway house, where he received good psychosocial rehabilitation and training as a food-service worker. The halfway house did not believe in therapy, so it was not offered. R.J. took medicine for several months; but he did not like to and he felt less depressed than he had, so he stopped taking the pills. Shortly after his training was over, he moved to the nearest large city with a gay community. He got a series of increasingly solid jobs in food service and was working in the most recent of these, some 20 years later, when the bus hit him.

R.J. had had two sequential long-term homosexual relationships, both with transvestite men substantially older than he was. The relationships were never faithfully monogamous. Although they had elements of real caring and mutual commitment, these coexisted with mutual exploitation and lack of faithfulness. R.J. cooked, did the housework, and catered sexually to the partners' preferences. They took care of the verbal, intellectual, and social tasks that R.J. could not handle.

Therapists can never really or fully be sure about such things, but my reconstructive sense is that this way of life was coming to an end for R.J. before—*shortly* before—the bus hit him. He was becoming older, less appealing physically, needier, and crankier, the festering needs beginning to surface. His job may soon have been obviated by a technological advance or may have been contracted out by the government agency for which he worked. His modest income over time was less and less of a contribution to his roommate. In addition, AIDS was changing everything, making both R.J. and his partner more cautious and less cautious at the same time ("Why put up with me if we're probably both going to die, anyway?"). Perhaps, as had been the case with the breakdown 20 years earlier, the accident was the inevitable product of a life course that needed to change direction, of tectonic shifts of unstable and unsatisfactory psychic structures and processes that sooner or later had to find a way to release. The injury was a product and a catalyst.

I have been working with R.J. for almost 5 years now. Some of the story is not worth telling—the workaday twists and turns, dry spells, and false starts. The work is slow and bumpy, in part because R.J. cannot tell me a straight chronology, keep out of trouble for long, or (yet) approach his intense bursts of feelings with the soothing and regulating perspective offered by self-awareness. Nevertheless, I have begun to notice some progress.

Therapy is characterized by a commitment to me listening to R.J.: He talks and I listen. Most people like R.J. never get access to this kind of long-term, in-depth therapy. Standard thinking would even advise against it, seeing R.J. as a poor candidate for either understanding the talk or acquiring significant insights. Yet the diagnostic picture and history I have been able to reconstruct are thorough, alive, and dynamic. They emerge from the therapeutic material of my sessions with R.J. and seem the best kind of proof that something of value transpires in the sessions and deepens over time. I can think of three other features that distinguish this therapeutic work as well.

First, much of what happens in the therapy happens in my mind, not R.J.'s. There is more containing than interpreting, and little press for insight. Similar to what Alvarez has suggested about the work of Bion (see Alvarez, 1992), R.J. projects fragments into me, and I may have to connect these into a meaningful pattern over a time frame of years before a clear enough thought would emerge for R.J. to take back into himself. This means that often the work is achingly dull and feels empty, as if I am seeking out the scraps of life in a psychic desert. Looking in at a therapy hour from the outside, an observer could easily think this was a supportive psychotherapy, distant from anything psychodynamic. But this is not the case; nor is the therapy devoid of movement.

Second, I am willing to take on concrete tasks. I have made phone calls, battled bureaucrats, and fought hard for 3 years for R.J. to get Social Security. Sometimes this flows from very basic pragmatic and moral concerns. No productive work can succeed if R.J. loses diabetic control or becomes homeless. But, more than this, work about concrete needs, done in the context of a therapeutic relationship, seems to expand the therapeutic field and potentiate its therapeutic properties, not constrict them. When R.J. and I negotiate how to battle "the system" together, even if I am doing more of the work than he is, what gets created is akin to a classic transference neurosis—a tangible re-creation of core issues in a way that is within range of mutual experience and discussion. When I take action on his behalf, outside the boundaries of conversation during the therapy hour, R.J. recognizes that there are things that he, as a person with significant physical, psychiatric, cognitive, and language disabilities, cannot do for himself. That reality needs to be present, articulated, and examined, as does the reality that the basic social safety net is grossly inadequate. If I cannot succeed in pulling strings for R.J., he will have to manage without. He has often gone months unable to get needed medicines. It will probably happen again. And yet these struggles for concrete necessities have had a cumulative impact, a kind of working through. R.J.'s life is now more ordered, his basis for survival more secure. And this is a basis for extending and deepening his therapeutic work.

Finally, I do not hold back from validating R.J.'s positive achievements and advances. I do not hesitate to tell him when I think he has made a good decision or approached a situation with a more mature or tolerant disposition. I have been influenced in this approach by Gardner's (1992) clinical findings that there are fewer "hard edges" in therapy than we used to think and that tactful, theoretically grounded psychoeducational elements will not necessarily annihilate therapy's dynamic properties.

In this sense I conceive of my work with R.J. as psychodynamic rather than psychoanalytic therapy. I'm not sure if he will ever develop enough cognitive, language, or ego capacity to engage in the work of deepening self-understanding for its own sake and on his own initiative. I may be proved wrong about this, and specifically wonder whether taking on the incest will open a way toward a more analytic feel to our work. I do notice a powerful response to judicious, attuned, occasional doses of positive feedback. Rather than infantilizing him, moments of guidance and validation seem to contribute to R.J.'s reservoirs of will and of courage, keeping him going in a line of work he approaches with serious handicaps.

~

R.J.'s progress is evident in several areas. He recently moved in with gay male friends, a couple, one of whom is ill with AIDS. His decision to live with friends rather than more disconnected roommates seems to reflect a recently and imperfectly acquired capacity to be more open emotionally—to want and be able to be with friends. His outbursts are also more controlled, so that friends—*good* friends—might be able to tolerate him as a roommate. The move, which we spoke about in an open-ended way, also represents R.J.'s willingness to participate in his friend's care, a need to give something back that, as we have examined it, seems at least in part to be genuinely sublimatory and altruistic.

R.J.'s family, including his son, hates him and will not see him. He hates them back for this and for many other reasons, but underneath he pines for their love or at least acceptance. Thus, when the brother who molested him made overtures toward contact, R.J. accepted them with equanimity and even a little excitement.

Outside the family, he has made some good friends. He is active in a gay fathers' organization and regularly attends a gay church, where he also takes American Sign Language classes. I see this as a transitional space in which he is working toward a more positive and integrated view of his own disabilities.

R.J. settled his case last summer. He got enough to pay off his debt to me and buy a car. He will also receive a small amount of money each month for the next 10 years. In addition, R.J. now receives Social Security disability, based on a bureaucratically sanctioned judgment that he is too disabled to be able to work. As soon as he got it, he found a job, which he held for several months before finding a better job. Securing this job was the culmination of R.J.'s willingness and desire to re-enter the work world. The satisfaction R.J. derives from working has been significant for him and may well lead him forward.

A CT scan confirmed my impression of a brain injury. Incredibly (but not really; such phenomena are common when persons with disabilities meet the medical system), the hospital where R.J. was brought after his accident had a plastic surgeon stitch his forehead anesthetically, but never thought to examine the brain that lay behind it. R.J. gets medicine for headaches and muscle spasms from a neurologist, and for biological depression from a physiatrist (he responded quickly and well, and psychiatric consultation has never seemed necessary or accessible). He is followed by a diabetologist and an orthopedist as well, and by an excellent physician assistant at a nonprofit clinic for the general medical care of people with disabilities. He has not recovered much function from surgery or physical therapy, but perhaps he will in the future. It has never been clear how much his bad attitude has constrained his recovery of function or problematic pain control. Perhaps, as therapy has more of an impact, his physical status will improve.

R.J. fell into a good social service system by accident 3½ years into our work together. An application to a service system with a long waiting list floated to the top when they got a grant to start a program for people who met R.J.'s profile—people with multiple disabilities, not retarded, and eager to work. A case manager helps him read his mail, pay his bills, seek out services, tolerate confusion and frustration, learn necessary skills on his job, and plan his life. They spend a lot of time together. The case manager helps mediate fights with friends and roommates and offers a lot of support. The program is slated to last for 3 years. It is unclear what will happen after that.

And R.J. is in love with a sweet, chubby, somewhat repressed and naive but good-spirited man almost 20 years younger, who lives in a small city 50 miles away. The exchange seems fair: The lover tolerates R.J.'s limitations and emotional unevenness, and R.J. provides a sense of excitement and adventure. The relationship is in its beginning stages. Sometimes R.J. seems as committed to not working on it or thinking about it as he is to having it work out; as a therapist, I wonder what this ambivalence portends for the relationship's future. Still, the pleasure and pride in R.J.'s voice as he talks about the relationship are authentic and unmistakable. I have seen relationships that have survived a lifetime on less.

My work with R.J. continues. It is in its middle stage. At times we bicker and fuss, like a couple who can take each other on in a way that can be a little raw because we fundamentally like, trust, and respect each other. I can interpret unconscious motives, and R.J. can tell me my carefully wrought constructions are unproductive and wrong. He rarely offers any words of acknowledgment or thanks; that comes in the doing, not the telling. But at times we are both awestruck at the changes he has made and revel for a brief moment in how different things have become for him.

R.J. joined the million people in New York in June 1994, celebrating the 25th anniversary of the Stonewall riot that initiated the modern gay liberation movement. He saved up his money, brought along his wheelchair for the march because he cannot walk distances, and had the time of his life. When he told me he never thought he would go to New York—221 miles from where he lives, and light years from where he lives psychically—I thought of how enraged and pessimistic I had felt about him in the beginning and how much that had changed.

I have no idea how much longer we will continue therapy. Perhaps, like many character-disordered patients, R.J. will reach a point where he is content with a still fairly symptomatic equilibrium. Perhaps our disabilities will themselves pose a constraint on the work we'll be able to do together. In the best scenario, we will make discoveries and integrations that neither one of us can yet imagine.

REFERENCES

Alvarez, A. (1992). *Live company*. New York: Tavistock/Routledge.

Gardner, V. (1992). Power and hierarchy: Let's talk about it. *Family Process, 32,* 157–162.

7

Sebastian

Comfort and Safety

Ann Steiner

I knew Sebastian for only the last 8 months of his life, but he was one of my greatest teachers. Our work began before there was much reliable information about AIDS, and therapists were just beginning to realize that to be gay was to live in a war zone. AIDS has had far-reaching effects on the gay community. Gays were surrounded by unremitting death, hostility, and physical violence on the streets. They also faced discrimination in the workplace, housing, and medical insurance. Medical care was too often inadequate. Patients and their partners were torn by the very real concerns about transmissibility. Weekends were now spent going to funerals and memorial services. This was a community under constant threat. Few therapists working with AIDS patients had experience negotiating the special demands of this debilitating, life-threatening illness. In addition, most therapists working in the gay community had little experience coping with the unique issues so common to individuals with chronic and life-threatening illness. Sebastian challenged me to become more flexible and creative. The exigencies of his life made it essential that both he and I take a more active role in his therapy than my training or the more traditional modes of treatment would allow. At the time, short-term therapy had not made its impact among private practitioners; yet much of the work we did together could now be considered brief focused therapy.

Although Sebastian could be described as a passive personality, and indeed had passivity problems with caretakers and others in his life, he could be quite directive in therapy. Early on, for example, he informed me that he didn't want to dig up early childhood issues or explore deeply his conflicts with people close to him. Although over time he was able to tolerate discussing his transference[1] feelings about me, he resisted examining the connection between his early life and current feelings toward me and his other caretakers. While there were times I found it difficult to follow his restrictions, I remember him with fondness and deep respect for his knowledge of himself—what he needed and what he could tolerate. His ability to state clearly where he wanted our work to go provided important guideposts in uncharted territory.

A 31-year-old Jewish gay man, Sebastian had been referred to me by a colleague for help coping with the pain and limitations caused by his Crohn's disease. The person who referred him felt that my work with Crohn's patients and patients with other chronic diseases made me a good match for him. Sebastian was also suffering from frequent bouts of thrush, chronic anal herpes, bronchial problems, and hearing loss from a collapsed eardrum. At the time I first saw him, he had not yet been diagnosed with AIDS. Within the first 2 months of therapy, however, he learned that he was HIV-positive and shortly thereafter found that he had full-blown AIDS.

The history of Sebastian's treatment can be divided into three phases, corresponding roughly to the phases of his physical condition. For each phase, I describe the therapy process, interspersing my description with commentary on the treatment.

~

Sebastian arrived 10 minutes early for his first appointment. He wore jeans and had a rumpled appearance. Tall and lanky, his demeanor was depressed and his face showed the effects of pain. He was being treated with antibiotics for his numerous infections and frequent bronchial problems, and clearly his Crohn's symptoms were taking their toll. He said that since he had been diagnosed with Crohn's, his life had changed drastically. Initially his employer had allowed him flexible hours, but recently he had been unable to work even part time at his job of office manager. He was tired of being sick, of going to doctors all the time, and distressed at feeling increasingly dependent on his roommate and others.

I inquired about his background, religion, and support systems. He described himself as a cultural Jew who grew up in an insulated, East Coast Jewish community, but he had never seen his religion as a

[1]Transference refers to feelings, desires, and emotional expectations from early childhood experiences that are later transferred to adult relationships. Transference to the therapist may be negative or positive. Understanding and resolving transference issues allows for emotional healing. As described later, the therapist's own transference reactions to the patient, countertransference, also must be explored by the therapist.

source of support. He was currently a member of a gay congregation, his membership paid by his roommate, Charlie, whom he described as an old college friend. Before beginning therapy with me, Sebastian had attempted to participate in several self-help groups with little success (with my encouragement, he was to join various other support groups during the course of our therapy). He had also had a brief, unsatisfactory experience with individual psychotherapy previously.

Sebastian's parents, sisters, and brothers all lived back East. He reported a new "closeness" with his family since he'd been diagnosed with Crohn's, but he did not elaborate. When asked about his childhood, he was guarded. He was willing to give me only a sketchy outline of his early childhood. He grew up witnessing much shouting and conflict between his parents—not a happy or emotionally nurturing home.

His years as a gay teen were "horrible." His first sexual experience occurred with a male friend at the age of 17. At the time, he did not think of himself as gay, and it wasn't until several years later that he began to identify himself as such. Shortly after his first sexual experience, he left a partially written love letter on his desk. His mother found it and showed it to his father, who went into a rage and beat him, calling him "disgusting" names. In passing, he mentioned that his father had had sex with him once. He would not elaborate on any of these episodes, insisting that he needed to focus on the present. Over time I learned that Sebastian felt that he had done all the repairing possible in his relationship with his family.

Sebastian showed up for his second appointment with his pants partially undone. He looked more disorganized and was more forgetful of the names of his medical team. He reported not feeling well. It was as though he needed to convey to me how distressed and out of control he felt. He complained that his knees hurt and relaxed noticeably after I offered him a footstool. As he became more relaxed, he spoke more freely about his feeling abandoned by the social worker assigned to him after his last hospitalization. He also complained of roommate problems, which he described in this session as "power plays."

Initially Sebastian had said he had been living for the last 2 years with an old college friend. But it now became clear that his roommate, Charlie, was a former lover and that they were currently nonsexual sleeping partners. In describing their relationship, Sebastian revealed an underlying passivity that I was to find typical in his personal relationships.

Therapist: Is this a love relationship?

Sebastian: Well, he ended up sleeping in my bed. In the beginning there was a little sexuality, but I soon lost interest. Then

> my sex drive got real low—I used to have it almost every day. Now I don't even feel affection. If I wake up next to him I get anxious and obsess about trying not to wake him. I don't feel warm toward him.

Sebastian characterized his roommate's attempts at intimacy (for example, tickling) as demanding. When I asked what his roommate could do differently, he was clear about what he wanted. He wanted to be asked questions, to have help offered without having to ask for it. He wanted to feel free to go to Charlie's room, tell him he was having trouble sleeping, lie next to him, be held, and not have to worry about "losing power." It is worth noting that with just gentle probing in therapy, Sebastian was able to be quite articulate about what would bring him comfort. The goal was to enable him to transfer this ability to his outside relationships, whether it was the intimate relationship with Charlie or more distanced ones with caretakers, without so much concern about power issues.

In passing, Sebastian mentioned that his last therapy had attempted to address his difficulties with intimacy. His intimacy problems would also be revealed by his ongoing ambivalence about another lover, Leonard, whom he had known 12 years before.

In a subsequent session we talked about his previous experiences with support groups and therapy. When asked about his experiences with the ileitis-colitis groups he had participated in, it turned out that he only ventured into the educational lectures, not the self-help support group: "I almost felt I wasn't sick enough, so I never went." Sebastian now felt sufficiently comfortable to talk about his previous therapy, which he referred to as "informal." He ended that therapy believing it would be too difficult to change the unsatisfactory way he and the therapist had worked together. He could not remember whether he had given the therapist any notice, except during the last session. He was able to see this as part of his pattern of not working things through in relationships. He was also aware of his difficulties with impulsivity.

When I encouraged him to schedule some termination sessions with his previous therapist, he was unwilling. His "stubbornness," as he called it, was fueled by the therapist's response: "I have a feeling you'll be back anyway." Sebastian responded to this as to a challenge: He would show him that he was different. He described feeling condescended to and admitted his anger at the therapist. He revealed that this therapist had talked about clients who had AIDS. The therapist had even described a visit with another patient who had dementia and had recently become blind. Although he had not had a diagnosis of AIDS at that time, this information terrified Sebastian. Clearly this prior therapist had major problems maintaining appropriate boundaries with his patient.

Not surprisingly, Sebastian preferred not to commit to a next appointment. We left it that he would call to schedule our next session. His numerous warnings about his sensitivity to power issues contributed to my decision to give him as much latitude as possible. I did, however, take the calculated risk of recommending that he seriously consider getting a medication evaluation. Specifically, I thought that some antidepressants might have the added benefit of providing some pain relief. Sebastian did request an antidepressant from his primary care doctor, and the Elavil prescribed for him provided significant relief. In addition, I urged him to make use of whatever support services and self-help groups were available to him. I explained to him that hearing from others coping with similar problems would reduce some of his isolation and could provide both practical and emotional support. I asked him if he would like me to speak to his primary care doctor as part of a team approach to his overall condition. With his consent, I was to talk with his physician and other caregivers several times over the course of the treatment. The results were generally productive.

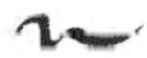

From the initial phase of therapy, a number of issues emerged that would be ongoing concerns throughout the treatment. From the little that Sebastian said about his childhood and family—and from much that he refused to say—it was evident that he had suffered early trauma. The glossed-over sexual incident with his father was the obvious example. This, as well as the verbal abuse and unmodulated anger in his home, contributed to a personality structure marked by distrust, struggles with passivity, and profound fears about taking action. The unprotected, unnurturing, anger-filled family situation was the source of his current complaints of indecisiveness, fear of intimacy, and inability to ask for help appropriately. Interestingly, Sebastian did not appear to be an overtly angry man, though from his history I would suspect hidden rage that he was very fearful of confronting.

If this were a less acutely ill person, I probably would have recommended long-term, in-depth, uncovering psychotherapy that would challenge his mechanisms for avoiding the painful past. However, he had his own urgent agenda. There were very pressing issues of physical losses, major lifestyle adjustments, and the current severe emotional trauma accompanying these losses. My decision to allow him to direct the therapy—to collude with his avoidance—was based at least in part on my feeling that it might be the only way to forge a therapeutic relationship.

My impression was that Sebastian was a frightened, skittish man, for whom trust was difficult. He was unable even to commit to a second appointment. To establish trust, I was willing to begin treatment with him on his own terms and to be more flexible with scheduling. This, I felt, would defuse his anxiety about control and powerlessness. He spoke vividly of seeing himself in a continual power struggle in which he was the loser (not unusual for patients with a history of abuse), and I felt that any authoritarian stance on my part would make a therapeutic alliance impossible. I was also convinced that I had to support that part of him that wanted to feel better, that was articulate about his needs, and that struggled for positive action.

During the first weeks of treatment, I discovered a contradiction between Sebastian's behavior with me and with other caregivers. While he was generally able to be direct, cooperative, and articulate about his needs in his sessions with me, he was unable to behave this way with his medical team, who perceived him variously as passive, helpless, needy, or aggressive. This first came to my attention when I spoke with his primary care doctor. I was surprised at the impatient tone in which his physician described Sebastian as overly concerned about his health, demanding, and whiny. Clearly the doctor was responding to this patient as if he were a hypochondriac. This is not an uncommon reaction of medical personnel when confronted with a patient with persistent, difficult-to-diagnose symptoms. I never saw him as hypochondriacal, however. Perhaps because of the therapeutic relationship, I was able to see his creativity and spunk, as well as his fears.

Initially, it was difficult for me to sort out how many of Sebastian's complaints were legitimate and whether he was creating further problems by the helpless, needy way he presented himself to caregivers. Over the course of our work together, I spoke with a number of his caregivers and members of his medical team. While they grudgingly conceded that he was having serious problems, I often found myself explaining Sebastian's emotional reactions and demands for greater information as necessary coping tools. I was able to help these overburdened caregivers to see Sebastian less as an irritant and more as a legitimately frightened man whose body was increasingly unreliable. It helped them to hear from me that he, too, was troubled by his excessive anxiety and was working hard in therapy to reduce it. Direct contact with his caregivers also helped me separate the medical problems Sebastian was responding to from the emotional ones. A primary goal of treatment was to keep his emotional problems from interfering with his obtaining the support, help, and information he required. We needed to transfer the behaviors he practiced successfully with me to his outside relationships.

The medically ill and other survivors of trauma often display a profound neediness that makes maintaining appropriate boundaries an ongoing challenge. There are many pitfalls to be avoided, such as a temptation to fight the patients' battles for them when they are capable of doing so for themselves; excessive distancing; or, as with Sebastian's previous therapist, inappropriate sharing of information and betrayals of confidence. Work with the medically ill requires that therapists be able to tolerate the trauma of patients' multiple fast-paced losses. The therapist's emotional responses to the patient's pain—countertransference (Reik, 1949)—is easily mishandled. Unless a therapist is finely tuned to his own countertransference reactions, damaging boundary violations are likely to occur.

Sebastian's neediness, his often forlorn and lost demeanor, evoked in me a desire to nurture him and to provide extra help—to lighten his burden. My countertransference was marked by my deep empathy for his fear of losing everything he had known and relied on. Each time I was confronted with a situation that made me feel I needed to take action to protect Sebastian, I reassessed the influence of my countertransference. With each variation from normal practice I had to ask myself whether I was doing his work for him. I analyzed my emotional reactions and reevaluated my motivations as well as the pros and cons of the action I was contemplating.

Sebastian's neediness led me to deviate from customary therapy boundaries in several ways. The first instance occurred after we had established a good therapeutic alliance. When he was too ill to meet with me in person, we tried a few phone sessions. Another nontraditional decision I made was to meet with him for double sessions when he hadn't been well enough to have a phone session. I felt that his need was legitimate and that my willingness to be more flexible was appropriate and useful under these specific circumstances. These accommodations allowed him to make use of his limited and fluctuating supply of energy when he had it.

A related departure from customary practice was my decision to work as closely as I did with his medical caregivers and later with his friends. I did so only after consulting with colleagues as well as with Sebastian to determine what was in his best interests. I always got Sebastian's input before talking to his caregivers, discussed what I had learned with him, and invited him to tell me how he felt about these contacts in an effort to make him an active decision maker in his own care. By collaborating with caregivers, I learned just how limited the resources available to him really were. I then felt freer to push him to be assertive with those who were most responsive and in a position to be of practical assistance. An additional benefit to this collaboration, although I could not know this at the outset, was that, having worked with his "team" throughout these months of illness, I was able to be a more effective advocate during his final hospitalization.

~

About 6 weeks after we started our work together, Sebastian became more ill. He suffered a return of his thrush condition, experienced greater joint and intestinal discomfort, and had more difficulty sleeping. At this time he learned he was HIV-positive. Sessions during this period were marked by his feelings of abandonment and frustration. He complained bitterly about his doctor's leaving town for 2 weeks. He was very fearful of not getting sufficient help and support and yet seemed to have great difficulty asking for help appropriately. At times, he wished he would get pneumonia. As we examined this wish, his fantasy of escape into a more serious illness that would assure him more intensive care and structure became clear. I encouraged him to look for other forms of relief. On my urging, he finally contacted the Shanti Project (a nonprofit, peer-based program that provides volunteers who offer practical and emotional support) and requested a volunteer to help him with chores in the home. At this time, he had also been seeing an acupuncturist for relief of chronic pain, and he needed to have our sessions scheduled around the acupuncture appointments. He had great difficulty requesting this of me. I wanted to encourage his efforts at self-care and was usually able to accommodate him. There were also numerous times throughout our work together when he called to reschedule our sessions so that he could be seen by his doctors on an urgent basis. I thought it was very important to encourage him to be more actively involved in his health care and to support his efforts to obtain medical information and any reassurance that would increase his comfort. At the outset, I made it clear that I would do my best to be flexible with scheduling and would tell him when I was not able to accommodate his schedule.

As we explored his options during the following days, he mentioned that his roommate, Charlie, had offered to take him to a resort for a weekend retreat. During the next few weeks of therapy, he continued to struggle with whether to take Charlie up on this offer. Sebastian was frustratingly vague about why he was ambivalent about taking this trip. After much probing, his many concerns became clearer. The trip involved a long airplane flight, and he worried about the medical risk of his eardrum bursting. Topping the list of logistical worries were the problems of finding bathrooms and getting a bed with sufficient support in the hotel. He also obsessed about whether to use a wheel chair in the airport. Using this aid represented for Sebastian, as it does for many other patients with disabilities, a distressing loss of mobility and power, as well as a social stigma.

The first task was to help him distinguish rational, reality-based concerns from his less rational fears. Having done that, he could then make his decision on a more informed basis. I took an active role in this process. I asked specific, detailed questions about the reality difficulties created for him by a change in environment. With each obstacle I invited his ideas and encouraged his creative problem solving. For instance, the thought of being pushed through the airport and having to ask someone to take him each time he wanted to go to the bathroom was humiliating to Sebastian. As we explored the issues, he concluded that being in the wheelchair would allow him to save energy better spent walking on the beach. To help him problem-solve, I told him about my Pain Price Index (see next page), a tool to assess which activities are most important to the individual, what they cost physically in terms of pain, symptom exacerbation, fatigue, recuperation time, and so on. Once the cost of a desired activity is spelled out, the patient can then decide whether it is worth the price.

In Sebastian's case, this problem-solving tool helped him decide whether the change in environment and the pleasures of beautiful scenery and fishing would be worth the likely necessity of 2 days of complete bed rest to recuperate. The result of this work was that Sebastian was for the first time able to view the trip as fun, a rare word in his vocabulary. And he was also able to consider the difficulties Charlie was facing in taking care of him. He began to talk with concern for Charlie's growing depression and decreased playfulness. His belief that the trip would give Charlie a lift was also a significant factor in his decision.

Sebastian finally risked traveling to the resort. He enjoyed the scenery, but fainted from heat stroke. He also came down with a serious cold. Nevertheless, he described his trip enthusiastically and said it had been worth the price.

Improving quality of life, reducing stress wherever possible, and taking breaks for relaxation and pleasure are treatment recommendations I make for most of my patients. However, for the medically ill, mobility impairments, pain, fatigue, and illness are serious obstacles to these goals, and problem solving requires great effort and creativity. Reality obstacles, practical dilemmas, and difficulty making decisions are typical, often daily, experiences for those with disabilities or illnesses. The Pain Price Index can serve as guide to making major and minor decisions, even when they must be subject to constant,

PAIN PRICE INDEX

Desired activities	Emotional benefits	Physical costs	Cost/Worth the price?
Gardening	Pleasurable outdoor activity. Feels like a contribution to family. Sense of competence and independence.	1 day of modified bed rest to recuperate plus no driving, typing, and cooking for 2 days.	Moderate/Worth the price once a month.
Sewing	Pleasurable activity. Feels like a contribution to self and family. Outlet for creativity. Sense of competence and independence.	2 days complete hand rest, or 1 day hand rest if sew only 10 min. every half hour.	Moderate/Worth the price twice a month. May require giving up activities with equal physical demands.
Vacuuming	Necessary for clean, healthy environment. Exercise. Feels like a contribution. Sense of independence.	3 days of pain and restricted mobility if more than 5 min. at a time.	Moderate/Not worth the cost. Decide to have children vacuum in exchange for help with their homework.
Dancing	Joyful activity, socially rewarding. Exercise.	5 days of pain and increased joint damage.	Severe/Occasionally worth the cost of pain since this level of enjoyment is rare.
Chopping wood	Pleasurable activity. Exercise. Contribution to family. Sense of competence.	5 days of pain, restricted activity, increased sleep disruption, unless done no more than 3 minutes at a time with frequent rests.	Severe/Worth the cost.
Washing dishes	Necessary chore. Feels like a contribution.	Several hours increased stiffness pain and swelling of hands.	Moderate/Worth the cost when no one else can do it.

sometimes hourly revision. We must encourage patients to allow for occasions when participation in an activity is worth the cost of the pain it engenders, now or later. Tools such as this index help patients find the proper balance between the benefit and the pain. Without finding this balance, or constantly working to build it, the patient will be trapped between the extremes of either overdoing things or never attempting meaningful activities.

Three months into treatment Sebastian's doctor informed him that he had AIDS. His immediate reaction was significant: "It's not terminal, but now I can get more Shanti services, free rides, and a home nurse to help." The relief evident in his response was understandable: his complaints, his need for help and sympathy, were now legitimized with the official diagnosis. He could no longer be considered hypochondriacal. Perhaps he would be listened to.

This reaction is typical of the relief experienced at the end of a long period of uncertain diagnoses. Most chronically ill patients have war stories to tell about the years of heartache and self-doubt that preceded their finally being awarded a diagnosis. Without a diagnosis that adequately explains their symptoms, patients often question the legitimacy of their experience. This complicates the already complex process of asking for help and coming to terms with increased dependency on others.

Relief, to be sure, is only one reaction, and Sebastian's relief was short-lived. He had begun to withdraw socially and described long periods of painful loneliness. For the first time, he began to imagine what it would be like to die. Even as his need for nurturance was heightened, he would only accept help from friends when it was offered rather than asking for it directly. The theme of whether he was sick enough to ask for help emerged in most issues we discussed.

For Sebastian, like most chronically ill patients, the firm diagnosis made it somewhat more "legitimate" to consider asking for help, but his personality structure and history still made it extremely difficult for him to do so. On inquiry, he revealed that he was "protecting" his friends by not asking for help. If they called, he'd ask for help; but during this time his friends weren't calling as often. I suggested that they might not know how they could help him without his letting them know directly. This was especially likely because he often turned down visitors when he felt unwell without arranging alternate times for visits. "Protecting" friends had complex meaning for Sebastian. He wished not only to protect his friends from the fear and distress of his illness but to protect them in the sense of preserving a store of friends. The fear and experience of being a burden is common. The chronic medically ill often fear that they will "use their friends up." These beliefs and assumptions must be explored and challenged.

Patients usually do have some friends who cannot tolerate the uncertainty and distress of being with an ill person (LeMaistre, 1993). It is very important to help patients determine who among their friends are the most willing to provide help and comfort and when to seek their help.

Among Sebastian's friends, the most important were Charlie and Martha. Charlie, his roommate, was certainly his best friend. He supplied emotional and physical support, and as the need increased he provided essential financial support as well. As Sebastian's health deteriorated, Charlie allowed him to live with him rent-free and paid his medical bills when his benefits were exhausted. Their relationship was intense and complex. Affectionate and caring on both sides, it was also marked by the anger, frustration, loss, and sorrow that are inevitable with the severe illness and decline of one partner. Their problems were exacerbated by Sebastian's underlying fears of intimacy, dependency, and loss of power.

Martha had been a close friend for several years. When Sebastian became ill, she was flexible and helpful in giving both physical and emotional support. She was very willing to take him to doctors' appointments and to chauffeur him around. She listened to him compassionately and was quite accepting and unthreatened by his physical and emotional problems. Although Sebastian at times found her physical affection for him uncomfortable—he perceived her touch as motivated by sexual attraction and experienced it as invasive—he was nevertheless very grateful to her, describing her as a nurturing, caring, steadfast person. Both Martha and Charlie remained pillars of support.

In contrast to these two was Leonard, a former lover about whom Sebastian had powerful feelings of longing mixed with anxiety. Unreliable and capricious, he nevertheless figured quite powerfully in Sebastian's fantasies, serving primarily as a distancing mechanism. Whenever Sebastian and Charlie began to get along better and feel closer, as during their weekend vacation, Sebastian responded to the increased intimacy by retreating into fantasies about Leonard.

Aside from Leonard, Sebastian was actually quite fortunate throughout his illness to have a small circle of close, caring, reliable friends. His difficulties with them stemmed from his problems asking for help, which arose directly from his history of abuse. Survivors of abuse often learn that it is dangerous to ask for help or to trust others. Although he refused to explore the origins of his problems, Sebastian was quite eager for practical suggestions to improve his relationships. I suggested that he establish an agreement with his friends: They would tell him frankly when they didn't have the emotional room to hear about his problems and would also let him know when they felt more available to him. He in turn would do the same for them. With great difficulty and many setbacks, Sebastian began to learn in therapy how to use this coping tool.

Patients must deal not only with their own relationships but with the disappointments and vicissitudes of the external world—the capriciousness of both government and private agencies and the not uncommon unreliability of even well-meaning caregivers. Sebastian, for instance, suffered painful feelings of loss and abandonment when a Shanti counselor canceled many meetings with no explanation. Such seemingly unreliable behavior engenders not only sadness and feelings of loss, but also anger. I encouraged Sebastian to talk directly with this counselor. I also suggested that there probably would be times when he was disappointed and angry with me. I emphasized how important it was that he let me know as soon as possible if he felt angry with me so that we could try to resolve the issues. He felt it necessary to assure me that he couldn't imagine ever feeling that way about me, but he did agree to let me know if such feelings did surface.

About halfway through our therapy, Sebastian experienced one of his brief upturns in physical comfort and stamina. Rather wistfully he reported that his home care had been discontinued because he no longer required nursing care. His home-delivered meals had been discontinued with his returning strength. Here Sebastian faced a dilemma common to the chronically or acutely ill—dealing with the very real threat of losing comfort, support, and structure with any improvement in physical condition. This dilemma reactivates anxieties about helplessness and the legitimacy of asking for help or comfort. Furthermore, patients often worry about the difficulties of reinstating previous levels of assistance, should their health again deteriorate.

When a physical condition changes, even for the better, grief and sadness over missed opportunities frequently flood the patient. Longed-for previously pleasurable activities are now possible, thereby eliciting a wide range of emotions that can be quite surprising and mystifying to a patient. Helping the individual understand this *improvement distress* allows further healing and integration. Some of the distress over "lost time" emerges at times of improved health since it can now safely come into consciousness. Once a patient is not completely absorbed with survival, longings for previously pleasurable activities resurface. Furthermore, recalibrating one's expectation of every daily activity is a daunting task. Everything previously known has to be reevaluated. While improved function is an exciting gift, this reevaluation process presents many new dilemmas that usually make patients feel painfully alone. The patient is the only one who can do this work of starting all over again. Caregivers, who are unaware of both the patient's sense of loss of support and structure and the emerging grief about lost time, are frequently mystified and disturbed by these reactions. Their common question is: "What's the matter—aren't you happy that you're better?"

I explained to Sebastian that his anxieties and increased indecisiveness were normal reactions to the loss of a known set of physical limits. I commented that starting over is always hard and suggested that we make coping with these changes a new short-term goal. Specifically, he needed to determine what options his body would now allow. For example, he had to figure out whether he could drive to appointments by himself, whether he could manage carrying his own groceries, whether he could risk being alone in the house when he took a bath. We explored each possibility systematically, prioritized the ones that were most important and decided on realistic and safe ways of testing his expanded limits. With my urging he had a telephone installed in the bathroom, which allowed him to feel more safe being there alone. He determined he was able to drive himself to several medical appointments and even to the beach a couple of times.

Unfortunately, his physical improvement was brief. Shortly thereafter, Sebastian called requesting an extra session. He was anxious because he had learned he would have to have his eardrum drained, a very painful procedure, and he worried about further hearing loss. It was not clear at this point if his concern was realistic, but I felt that his ability to request an extra session was a sign of progress. At this time he began to report problems with driving, sleep disturbance, grogginess, and frequent fevers. His depressive stance came into sharper focus, as he responded to his physical setbacks with profound feelings of hopelessness and fear about increased dependence on others. An issue that resurfaced at this time was his distress and anger at his primary care doctor, who, frustrated and impatient with Sebastian's neediness, had admonished him: "You can't come in every time you have a fever; you have to figure out which fevers require medical attention."

Always for Sebastian the issue of recognizing and defining realistic boundaries was critical. He frequently seemed unable to find an appropriate middle ground between reluctance or inability to seek information and help and an overdemanding, pestering attitude with caretakers. His doctor, even if impatient, was attempting to set realistic boundaries with his patient. One solution I suggested was for us to devise a list of questions to ask at his next medical visit: What can I eat? Are the bowel problems symptoms of AIDS or Crohn's disease? What about drug interactions?—and so forth. He did, in fact, present a one-page list of questions to his doctor, who responded positively to this approach and was able to provide answers to several of his concerns.

I also urged Sebastian to continue to seek more varied support for some of his problems through participation in adjunct support groups. A relaxation or meditation group could be of great value in relieving his sleep disorder, and an AIDS support group would reduce isolation and be a safe place for shared problem solving. This was critically important for Sebastian. He badly needed to realize that he himself had something to offer others.

The timing of referrals to adjunct support groups for patients who are feeling traumatized and who have suffered multiple losses requires careful consideration. This is especially true for people who are isolated and feel that their connections to others are tenuous. They may interpret any referral to outside groups as rejection. The medically ill are at greater risk of interpreting these referrals to mean that their neediness has overwhelmed the therapist. When we explored this issue, Sebastian did admit to some anxieties about my referrals to these groups, but he felt that the benefits of such outside help outweighed his fears, and he did begin to participate in a meditation group and an AIDS support group.

Actually, Sebastian had dabbled in such groups before but characteristically had fled when issues became difficult. The challenge was getting him to stick with them. One incident was typical. When his hearing worsened, he simply stopped going to his AIDS group without telling the group leader that he could no longer hear the other members. It hadn't occurred to him to ask his group leader to set up a small amplifier in the room to make his continued participation possible—a simple, inexpensive technical solution to his problem. Sebastian needed steady encouragement to stay committed and connected to these support groups.

About 4 months into treatment, I met with Charlie. Quite early in therapy Sebastian had asked me to do so. I was willing to consider a meeting, but only after we had explored thoroughly why he wanted me to meet Charlie and what his expectations of such a meeting would be. His reasons were exposed over time. At first he said he wanted me to understand his home life: "What I'm up against." His complaints about Charlie were superficial—his lack of humor, his compulsive neatness. As I probed, Sebastian's real reason for wanting me to intervene with Charlie emerged—his fear of abandonment by him. In this fear was projected his own anger at his illness and at himself. He wished me to "safeguard" their relationship by encouraging Charlie to resume his own individual therapy. At the same time Sebastian was greatly fearful of a very real possibility: that if Charlie did resume therapy, his therapist might encourage him to break off his relationship with Sebastian.

Certainly their relations were becoming increasingly tense. What should have been negotiable issues began to take on huge importance. A case in point was Charlie's offer of a VCR. It became a symbol of Sebastian's difficulty accepting help without feeling intolerably indebted and powerless. Charlie was understandably hurt at being considered a "power monster" for offering an aid that would bring comfort and relaxation to both of them. It took several sessions to clarify and defuse Sebastian's concerns before he finally accepted this gift.

From what Sebastian had been saying about their increasing difficulties, I agreed with him that a meeting with Charlie would be useful; and once Sebastian's expectations were clarified and explored, I scheduled a meeting with his roommate. It came at a critical time. Their difficulties had come to a head when, in a seemingly ordinary quarrel, Charlie's own suppressed anger finally exploded, and he asked Sebastian to leave. Sebastian was wounded and responded by placing calls for emergency housing. Although the incident blew over in a day or two, it was clear that Charlie and Sebastian were suffering acutely.

My session with Charlie revealed how close to reality Sebastian's fears were. Charlie's depression and grief were obvious. He described being unable to control his crying at work, and he had severe conflict about staying with Sebastian rather than accepting a promotion in another city. He felt imprisoned by his commitment to Sebastian, yet he also described it as "a nice prison." He was not at all sure whether he wanted anything to change. I told him I thought it a mistake for him to take care of Sebastian physically, that that role could best be filled by either privately hired help or agency staff. This would allow them to maximize the more positive qualities of their relationship. His fear that therapy would melt the last of his denial was palpable. As we talked about his pain, he came to see that he, like Sebastian, was in need of support. I encouraged him to resume individual therapy to deal with his anger and depression and to join a caregiver's support group, which he eventually did. He commented that our session had been useful to him. It was useful to us both in that it helped establish a working alliance that was increasingly important as Sebastian became more ill.

~

In the following weeks I noticed what I feared was a deterioration in Sebastian's cognitive functioning, as well as in his physical condition. Two incidents brought this to my attention. Sebastian had called me in a panic. He had just spent 7 hours in a mattress store unable to choose a comfortable mattress. He was extremely distressed at his inability to make a decision and was overwhelmed with the feeling that there was "no comfort anywhere." Only after he postponed his mattress hunt for the time being did his panic and depression abate. A few weeks after this phone call, the weather turned cold and Sebastian decided he needed the "right" raincoat. He had finally selected one he liked, but once he got it home found a minor problem that he considered unacceptable. His reaction to this disappointment was as intense as his panic over the bed. He then made a connection between his indecision about the bed and his disappointment about the raincoat: "This might be the bed I'll die in and the last raincoat I'll own." Although his sentiments were understandable, his increased panic and depression had a different tone to them that made me suspect organic involvement.

Concerned, I called his primary care physician. He told me Sebastian was rapidly deteriorating from the "worst kind of AIDS," wasting encephalopathy. The doctor reported that Sebastian was calling the office excessively and attributed this to a combination of short-term memory loss and "denial." He warned me to expect more deterioration: "His deterioration will continue until he is a bedridden vegetable. He has, at the most, 6 months to live. In the meantime, he's a lost soul." I asked how much of what I was currently seeing was organic. He confirmed that there was significant organicity combined with what he referred to as Sebastian's "passive personality style."

I asked the doctor if he had been as direct with Sebastian about his condition as he had been with me. He said that he had told Sebastian that he should no longer leave home alone, but he had not been completely frank about the gravity of his condition, preferring to let him cling to hope. Sadly, Sebastian's lifelong problem of having his experience invalidated was once again unwittingly reinforced by his physician. Sebastian knew he was deteriorating, yet his doctor was not prepared to confirm this reality. As we talked further, the doctor decided now was the time to tell him. That same day he met with Sebastian, told him frankly about his condition, and suggested that he begin to use hospice services.

I was now treating not a chronically ill patient, but a terminally ill one. Sebastian now faced a new set of painfully difficult tasks—he would have to confront and prepare for his own death. As a therapist, I would have to help him do this. I, too, would have to confront his death and prepare myself for it.

Sebastian responded to his prognosis with a mixture of relief, rage, anxiety, and depression. Not surprisingly, his old conflicts about dependency, trust, abandonment, and control came into play as he began to prepare for his own death. These conflicts made it even more difficult to make necessary end-of-life decisions. I felt that an important part of my role as a therapist was to point out which of these decisions he was not dealing with and to encourage him to do so as a way of making things easier on himself.

The most pressing issue was to determine what to tell his family and how much to involve them in this final phase of his life. Sebastian was able to tell his mother and sister that he was dying. Although he appreciated their offers to have him live with them, he was, as the result of our work, able to make the decision he felt was best for him—to remain in the community of friends that he had created. This involved not only refusing the aid of his family, which was a sad decision for him, but putting to rest some of his ungrounded mistrust and fear that Charlie would abandon him.

The next urgent issue was for Sebastian to make legal arrangements: for power of attorney, for durable power of attorney for health care decisions, and for dispersal of personal property and life insurance. I encouraged him also to take charge by planning his memorial service, and the idea of being in control of this last ritual appealed to him. Dealing with these complex matters, however, was doubly difficult because of his AIDS-related brain damage. It became increasingly difficult to sort out personality problems from cognitive impairment. I had to repeatedly push him to resolve issues that interfered with his making decisions. He obsessed continually, for instance, about how to divide up his personal property and assets. If he left everything to Charlie, then his family would feel slighted. If he left only half to Charlie, how could he divide the rest of it fairly? If Charlie found out he was only to get half of Sebastian's assets, maybe Charlie would kick him out. Because of his organicity I had to take on a more active, structuring role than previously and continually reality-test with him. Before his final hospitalization, however, we did manage to settle these legal issues.

About this time Charlie called, sadness slowing his speech. Sebastian hadn't been lucid for several days and would have to be hospitalized. I next saw Sebastian in the acute care unit. With his hospitalization my role once again shifted dramatically. My collaborative work increased. I became his emotional advocate, working actively with his hospital staff, who found his behavior very trying. I asked that my phone number be listed in his hospital chart so that staff could contact me when he became agitated. The next day his nurse called to tell me that he had been calling his doctor every 5 minutes and asked that I talk to him. My call, which lasted less than 10 minutes, made him feel less frightened and alone. It was to be the first of many. Other staff soon became comfortable calling me for advice on how to calm him. During the next few weeks, I visited Sebastian frequently. He often asked me to hold his hand, which I did. The dementia was winning. Terror and paranoia were taking over. Sebastian needed constant reassurance that his food was not being poisoned, and he turned with suspicion from most of his friends.

The environment he now lived in was a shock to me. His hospital room was filled with several large cans printed with enormous red letters and the poison sign. The word *contamination*, although unspoken, was written everywhere. It felt like a leper colony. Most hospital rooms are impersonal and somewhat dehumanizing, but this went beyond anything I had yet experienced. Sebastian's lips were chafed and cracked. I applied Vaseline swabs and gave him ice sticks to relieve his painfully dry mouth. I and the few friends and family members who stuck with him to the end were the only ones who approached his hospital bed without gloves, masks, and surgical gowns. In this bizarre setting, I fought my own demons to maintain the emotional connection he had allowed me the honor of sharing. It was painful to watch him waste away, and I needed to allow myself time after my visits with him to recover and regroup before going back to my other world.

On Charlie's request and with his therapist's encouragement, I met with Charlie once while Sebastian was in the hospital. In this session and in the numerous brief contacts we had in the hospital, we talked of his grief and the trauma of watching this plague destroy his best friend. I was able to remind him of Sebastian's feistiness, playfulness, and strengths. At one time when Charlie was tempted to jump ship, I talked with him about the deeper intimacy the two of them had shared over the last year and encouraged him to take time to care for himself. I let him know that I realized staying connected with someone in the forbidding environment of the hospital, knowing he was dying, was no easy task. At times I was the only one capable of seeing how much a gift Charlie's visits were to Sebastian.

A few days after my last hospital visit, Charlie called to say that Sebastian had died. Both he and Martha made it very clear that it was important to them that I attend at least the memorial service. Being invited to this service was one of the most difficult dilemmas I had yet faced. My psychoanalytic training clearly prohibited any such crossing of boundaries. Yet my work with Sebastian had required that I leave these strictures behind long ago. I was forced to sort out my countertransference reasons for going or not going. My main concern was what my role would be at the service: Could I balance my impulse to be an unfettered mourner with my professional role? I decided that closure was important to me as well as to them and that I would attend without participating in the service.

It was deeply moving to be included in the memorial rituals Sebastian had planned for his friends and family. Following the service, Charlie introduced several close friends to me, saying I was the one who had also served as a healer to Sebastian's community. People thanked me for urging Sebastian to accept help from them; they appreciated being able to make his life a little easier and more comfortable. It was comforting to be among those who loved and cared for Sebastian. It helped us all complete our goodbyes to this sweet, gentle soul.

> We are a peaceful loving people,
> And we are fighting for our lives,
> Fighting for our lives.
>
> —Holly Near

REFERENCES

LeMaistre, J. (1993). *Beyond rage: Mastering unavoidable health changes.* Oak Park, IL: Alpine Guild.

Near, H. Singing for our lives. On *Lifeline.* (Available From Redwood Records, P.O. Box 10408, Oakland, CA 94610.)

Reik, T. (1949). *Listening with the third ear: The inner experience of a psychoanalyst.* New York: Farrar, Straus and Company.

8

Individuals with Disabilities in Families and Society

An Empowerment Approach

Paul B. Feuerstein

This chapter describes therapeutic work with several persons with disabilities at Barrier Free Living, Inc., an agency founded in 1978 as a federally funded research and demonstration project of the Federation of the Handicapped. The project, founded for "homebound-prevention," provided prevocational intervention and vocational evaluation and training to persons with newly acquired disabilities. Early in its work, the project discovered that simply providing prevocational and vocational services was not sufficient. It began to expand its services to individual, family, and group counseling as well as individual and public advocacy. At the end of the federal funding, the project became a separate agency and expanded its mission to include all persons with disabilities and their families. While the agency provides mental health support, involving consumers in both personal and community advocacy has been a key ingredient in many of our successful rehabilitations.

Working with single persons with disabilities is complex enough. Working with persons who live with family becomes extremely complicated. Besides dealing with the coping process of the individual with the disability, the therapist must appreciate the coping process of each family member as well. Family members can provide major support for the person with the disability and create major barriers to rehabilitation—often at the same time. Many acts of good intention can create unneeded dependencies in which both the individual and the family become firmly invested.

The role of the person with the disability in the family prior to the onset of the disability as well as the roles that family members have assumed to adjust to the change in the family system are important factors to examine. The ability to problem-solve and the clarity, directness, and sufficiency of communication are also key factors.

Let us first define "family." Very few of the individuals who come to us for services fit the statistical norm of the nuclear family. We work with many single parents whose spouses without disabilities have abandoned the family. In other cases we work with couples who, because of medical or personal reasons, have decided not to have children. We have also, at times, treated the care attendant as a member of the family unit. Often a person with a disability has a closer working relationship with a care attendant than with any member of the family. This is particularly true when the attendant lives with the home care consumer.

Because almost all of the families we have worked with fall under the federal guidelines for poverty, an important external factor must be considered: the bureaucracy that must be negotiated in order to obtain shelter, food, medical care, and subsistence level income. These systems are usually more dysfunctional than the family systems we treat. The following cases illustrate the complexities that often lead to years of frustration but occasionally to success. I have chosen to discuss cases that are not classic family therapy situations but that capture some of the unique dynamics practitioners may encounter in working with persons with disabilities and their families.

Arthur and Madge came to us for help because Arthur's Parkinson's disease had progressed to a critical point. They came for financial advice and support, but other pressing issues also needed attention. Arthur was 54 years old and had had a successful career in the publishing business. His wife was 10 years his junior and had been satisfied as a homemaker. They reported that they had been happily married prior to the beginning of his Parkinson's disease. At the point when they sought help from us, he was no longer able to work and they were quickly depleting their life savings to support themselves and to pay for his medical care. His firm had allowed him to work on a part-time basis and had sent work to his home when he was no longer able to make it to the office, but his condition had deteriorated and this arrangement was no longer viable. They came seeking help to address the serious financial problems facing them. What we found was a couple that was becoming increasingly dysfunctional because of the changes in their roles and their physical and emotional inability to communicate. Madge had to suddenly assume the job of managing the family finances. Arthur had lost the ability to speak clearly, and Madge had taken up the task of being his interpreter to the world.

I found in Arthur and Madge a dynamic that often occurs in a family in which a member can no longer communicate clearly. This can be the result of aphasia secondary to a stroke or from a traumatic brain injury or the result of deterioration, as in Arthur's case. The contract that develops in the family in which one member becomes translator for another ultimately leads to a fused type of relationship. When Arthur and Madge would come in for a session, I would ask Arthur how he felt that day. Madge would answer, "He feels fine," or "He had a bad day yesterday." When I asked Madge how she was feeling, she was often at a loss for words to describe her own internal life. It became increasingly apparent that Madge both resented the role that she was trapped in and was invested in continuing that role out of a sense of obligation to her husband, reinforced by their shared religious values.

We began by addressing their presenting problem, for which there were no easy solutions. To qualify for the medical help that was needed, Arthur and Madge had to meet certain income and resource qualifications. We worked to prepare them for the time when such applications would be possible, once their resources were further depleted. In the meantime, they presented the need for supportive therapy to deal with their sense of loss and to strengthen their marriage. The enmeshed relationship was based on the very real difficulties of communicating with the outside world; thus, Arthur needed immediate assistance to help him build his skills of independent communication and to assist Madge in letting go of that role. I promptly involved Arthur and Madge in a group that included other couples and single individuals with recently acquired disabilities. One basic rule of the group was that members had to speak for themselves and for no one else. At first, this was a very uncomfortable position for Arthur and Madge. Arthur remained silent, with Madge hovering over him in a protective mode. Neither contributed much to the group. The group itself allowed that to happen for about a month before members began to ask Arthur about his opinions, experiences, and feelings. Madge immediately jumped in to answer for him, but she was reminded by group members that Arthur needed to speak for himself. It was a difficult and embarrassing venture for Arthur to make, but the group had other members who also had expressive problems. With each individual, a different set of accommodations was worked out. Arthur began—over a period of weeks—to express himself. Both he and the group got a great deal of satisfaction out of the experience. However, it was clear that Madge was not at all supportive of this direction. She expressed her disapproval through facial expression and body language. As she was challenged by the group, it came to light that Arthur's new-found skills were another source of loss in Madge's life. Arthur had a much easier time striking out toward independence than Madge had of letting go of her role as protector. Once she was able to articulate what was happening, we were able to begin the work of Madge developing her own agenda for her life apart from being Arthur's protector. Arthur gave her permission to move out of the role of translator/protector. Once she gave herself permission to do other things, the underlying level of resentment gave way to a new-found pride in her own accomplishments. This led to improved levels of communication between the two. They ceased doing couples' therapy when Madge went to work, and a care attendant was hired to take care of Arthur's needs.

~

The presence of a care attendant in the home often complicates the relationships between family members. New York's personal care regulations do not allow the care attendant to do any functions for other members of the family. On a policy level that makes sense, but on a day-to-day living level it creates many problems. A care attendant cooks for a parent with a disability. Who cooks for the child? A care attendant is responsible for cleaning the dishes of the personal care consumer. Whose dishes are in the sink? While many home attendants will participate in the informal give-and-take that facilitates the working of a family unit, many stick to the letter of the regulations, at times not even providing for the services needed by the personal care consumer. Many consumers are reticent if not fearful about challenging care attendants because of their dependency on the care attendants for activities of daily living. The level of negotiation necessary becomes overwhelming for the family unit.

Daniel was transferred to me by a worker leaving the agency. He was a 39-year-old Latino man with cerebral palsy and severe asthma who used a motorized wheelchair for mobility. He was somewhat overweight and had severe scoliosis. He also had alternating exotropia, an eye condition that made his right or left eye diverge from his focal point. This made regular eye contact with Daniel a challenge. I was never sure which eye he was using and whether he was maintaining eye contact or looking away from me. Although he had not finished high school because of a problem with mathematics, he was a highly articulate individual who had been an active advocate in the organized community of people with disabilities in New York. He was active in advocacy for accessible transportation. He participated in a suit against the Metropolitan Transit Authority that led to the requirement that all buses be wheelchair-accessible and to the implementation of a plan to make key subway stations accessible. He was active in personal care attendant issues and had strong feelings about the way the program should work for people with disabilities. His own relationship with his care attendant, however, did not correspond with his own public advocacy positions.

During the time I worked with Daniel, I sensed a great resistance to change. The image I have of Daniel is that of a large rock off the southern coast of Martha's Vineyard near my family's summer home. The waves crash against that rock every day, yet the rock never moves. Despite the way he has been personally attacked in his interpersonal relationships as well as in his vocational and educational life, he continues to remain the same. There were times during therapy when I challenged him about his commitment to change. He would smile and say the things he thought I wanted to hear but continued to be impenetrable, like that rock off the coast of Martha's Vineyard. There were many times when I felt he was using therapy as a means of providing emotional release without having to commit to change.

About a year before he started working with me, he had been in a car accident when he was riding in the street in his chair. The accident, which was not serious, threw him into a severe depression. He left his wife, who had more serious disabilities than he, and prior to beginning therapy with me, he had already been in two abusive relationships with women who had fewer disabilities than he did. The longest relationship he had was with his 24-hour-a-day care attendant. They had been together for 12 years. When questioned about the amount of time his care attendant usually spends with him, Daniel reported that she spends between 2 and 3 hours a day in his house. This suits Daniel's lifestyle because he feels the need for space in his relationships. When he is acutely ill and needs more service, his care attendant stays with him. (It is not unusual for individual consumers to work out their own arrangements with care attendants. Usually, however, the arrangements are not this extreme.)

In each of Daniel's relationships, he found himself torn between loneliness and wanting to be uninvolved with women. The easiest relationship for him was the one with his home attendant because she was on the payroll and was happy to be paid for 24-hour-service while providing less. At the same time this created tensions within his relationships with other women.

When he began working with me, Daniel was involved with Beatrice, a homeless woman. Daniel had invited Beatrice and her daughter to move in with him until she could find permanent housing. Daniel reported that he was emotionally and physically abused by Beatrice and that he wished for the relationship to come to an end. However, when Beatrice informed him that she was getting her own apartment, Daniel had very conflicted feelings about the move. He had come to depend upon Beatrice to help him with money management. Due to a learning disability, he had never been able to balance his checkbook. Even after Beatrice moved out, she had control over Daniel's money. Daniel and I spoke of his ambivalence and worked toward his becoming independent from Beatrice. Daniel swore off relationships and vowed to focus his attention on vocational issues. Daniel continued to experience very mixed feelings about breaking off the relationship with Beatrice and maintained contact with her.

About 6 months after Beatrice left, Daniel began a relationship with Pam, a woman he had met in a sheltered workshop that he had been placed in as part of his vocational evaluation. Pam had been a long-term participant in the sheltered workshop. She was slightly younger than Daniel and had a visual impairment. I wondered whether she was in the sheltered workshop because of the visual impairment or because of her intellectual functioning. In my first observations of her, she tended to see the world in very black and white terms, with little tolerance for subtlety.

Within 3 months, they were living together. At that point, I suggested couples' therapy to address the problems I saw arising in the relationship. Shortly after moving in, Daniel received a call from his ex-wife asking for help in finding a new care attendant. Daniel arranged for Pam to become her attendant. At the same time, Daniel and Pam allowed a series of transient individuals to live with them, cutting down on the time they had together and taxing their already limited resources. Pam's second job had already cut the amount of time they could spend together to a minimum.

Every one of these complications could be attributed to outside influences, but each one served to create distance between the two of them. These fit Daniel's pattern of creating space in relationships by using other people as buffers. After 5 months of couples' work, I was able to get Daniel and Pam to look at the problems with boundaries in their relationships. We worked together on learning limit-setting skills. Ultimately, Pam gave up her position with Daniel's ex-wife, and the couple worked on evicting the last of the transients who had come to live with them. The main unresolved issue was the relationship between Daniel, Pam, and Emily, Daniel's long-term care attendant. Pam was extremely angry with the situation within the household. She had gone through personal care training and knew what Daniel's care attendant was supposed to do for him. When Emily would not follow through on her responsibilities, Pam would jump into the situation with a great deal of anger and either cook, clean, do dishes, or otherwise care for Daniel. Within the context of a living-together relationship, everything Pam did was fairly ordinary. However, she resented Emily's being paid for the work that she was doing. Daniel's response to Pam's anger was to laugh it off. He stated that Pam should leave the dishes or the cleaning until Emily got around to it, but Pam refused to live in the level of disorder that Daniel was proposing.

At this point, I attempted family therapy sessions with the three of them. There was a great deal of resistance on Daniel's part to involving his care attendant in his therapy with Pam. Daniel's relationship with Emily was long-standing. It had served as a buffer for Daniel in his previous relationships with women. Prior to being in therapy, Daniel reported that he had been through a series of short-term relationships. The deciding factor in the dissolution of all of them was Daniel's relationship with Emily. I had no sense of any kind of romantic ties between Daniel and Emily. She had a husband and children in the suburbs and her 2- to 3-hour-a-day responsibilities fit well with her family life. All of the women in Daniel's life had difficulty with how little support Emily provided Daniel and how much Daniel became dependent upon them.

We attempted to address that issue within the family therapy sessions. This triangulated relationship created unique dynamics within the household. The longer, stronger relationship was between Daniel and Emily—with Pam being the newcomer. On one level Pam was friendly with Emily, and they had formed an alliance over some mutual issues with Daniel. However, they were never able to resolve the issues over Daniel's care. Daniel was resistant to having anyone else make suggestions about his relationship with Emily. He had very strong political feelings about the control a consumer should have over his personal care attendant. This became a screen by which Daniel could fend off solutions that came from either Pam or me within the context of our sessions. Emily was very clear that she worked for Daniel and would do whatever Daniel wanted. The crux of the problem was that Daniel was not sure himself of what he wanted.

When many of the obstacles that caused Daniel and Pam to be separated were overcome, they found new obstacles to get in the way. Daniel discovered that he liked talking to individuals on his new citizens band (CB) radio. We were also able to get him into a specialized college program that earned him his high school diploma as he was taking freshman courses. All of these things created distance between them. This finally led Pam to decide that she wanted to leave Daniel. Daniel was by this time uncomfortable with the relationship. His way of getting out was to create an untenable situation and wait for Pam to leave.

In addition to the conjoint sessions, I met with Daniel on an individual basis. He began to talk about his childhood. Daniel was raised by an alcoholic mother. He never knew his father. His father allegedly died when he was young. When Daniel was 12, his mother married again and had two more sons. Daniel reported that one is a drug addict and the other is in prison. His mother divorced his stepfather when Daniel was 20. Daniel's mother married again and had a daughter by her third husband. Daniel reported that he was never close to any of his siblings. He had gone to special schools and had returned home to an empty house every day. He spent most of his time in his own room. When he was 18, he went through a series of operations to correct his spinal problems. At that point his mother "abandoned" him and he dropped out of school.

His mother was employed as a medical secretary in a hospital. Daniel stated that he had always wanted to be a doctor. Given his learning disability and his not finishing high school, he began to recognize that this was an unrealistic goal. As we talked about his vocational goals, he vacillated between working in a sheltered workshop or as a television repairman, an actor, a public advocate in the political arena, or in some other position in which he would be recognized.

Daniel was a study in ambivalence. He wanted a relationship because he was lonely, but he feared being close because he would lose his autonomy. He wanted to be a leader of the disability movement, but he did not want the demands that come with leadership. He wanted to be in charge of his life, but he wanted to be taken care of. A combination of being the child of an alcoholic and an adult with a developmental disability created a set of life circumstances that led to entropy. However, after years of therapy, Daniel finally began taking steps to develop his vocational life. Daniel decided to go to college full time and has put both therapy and relationships on hold for a while. We have left the door open for him to return if he chooses to.

~

There are situations in which the dynamic of the disability can have a profound impact on a family unit. For individuals with severe disabilities who must depend upon social systems for survival, the dysfunction of the helping system can negatively affect the family dynamics. This may require the therapist to take on much more of an advocacy role to address the family's problems. Lengthy hospitalizations can cause long-term problems when small children do not have regular access to a parent.

Eliza came to our center with a complex set of problems. A 35-year-old African American woman with a left below-the-knee amputation secondary to juvenile-onset diabetes, Eliza was a tall, naturally graceful woman with attractive features. She was articulate and direct, choosing her words carefully. She was referred by a family protection agency, whose mission was to provide case management services to keep children out of foster care. Eliza's son had been hospitalized twice when he was 8 years old after claiming he had been hearing voices and seeing monsters. He had killed the family cat and hid it under his bed, where it had remained until the neighbors complained about the smell. When he was 9 years old, he allegedly set fire to their apartment. By the time I had begun working with Eliza, her son was 10 years old and was in Manhattan Children's Psychiatric Center.

Eliza was born in South Africa to a father who had seven wives and "countless" children. At an early age, Eliza moved to Florida with her mother and grandfather. Her grandfather died shortly thereafter, and Eliza moved to Virginia with her mother, two brothers, and two sisters. She had her first child, a daughter, when she was 14 and her first son when she was 15. She thought it would be fun to have children but found it difficult. Eliza was in prison briefly, for a crime she refused to discuss and her children were put in foster care. She had no contact with her children until they were 16 and 15, respectively. By that time, she had had her second son, Adam, who was diagnosed with schizophrenia. Adam as a baby had a number of significant separations from his mother due to her medical complications. Eliza's pregnancy with Adam triggered a loss of control of her diabetes, leading to many medical complications. When Adam was 3, Eliza was hospitalized for a protracted period of time for the amputation of her left leg. Adam was in foster care for that period of hospitalization. When he returned, he seemed to be stable, but a change in day care triggered his acting out in school. His performance continued to deteriorate, and he was placed in a special school for children with emotional disorders. During play therapy, Adam was reportedly preoccupied with feelings that his mother was dying or already dead.

Shortly thereafter, Eliza's two older children came to New York requesting to live with her. Eliza could not maintain control over either of them. Both children dropped out of school. Her daughter was described in a child protection agency report as "a disorganized, impulse-ridden retarded girl who had been psychotic in the past." She ran away from home and returned 2 years later to abduct Adam. She kept him for 4 days. He was reportedly the victim of sexual abuse during that time. At the time of our starting to work together, Eliza had just come out of the hospital after an amputation of part of her other foot. She was acutely depressed with hypersomnia as a primary symptom.

The main focus of Eliza's concern was the welfare of her child. It was clear that she was overwhelmed by her family situation, which had led to her voluntarily placing Adam in a psychiatric inpatient facility. My intervention began by setting up both individual and family sessions to build up Eliza's parenting skills and to help her cope with the loss of part of her other foot. As a result of her feeling overwhelmed by her present situation, she had withdrawn from both family and friends. We worked on an individual basis three times a month and had a family session with Adam at the Manhattan Children's Psychiatric Center once a month.

From the very first session, I could see Adam's overwhelming need for his mother and Eliza's overwhelmed response. Adam was an attractive young boy with big bright eyes and an appealing smile. He was tall for his age. He was generally dressed well and appropriately groomed, but his mother was not satisfied with his appearance or his grooming. His behavior was consistently characterized by high levels of distractibility, hyperactivity, and an extremely short attention span. He was usually in constant motion. He was also diagnosed with a learning disability.

Adam liked to sit in his mother's lap or to constantly hover around her, playing with her hair or patting her head. The more Adam clung to his mother, the more Eliza withdrew. In subsequent sessions, we dealt with her feeling overwhelmed by his advances and her efforts to fend him off, which were often interpreted as rejection.

We found that Adam best expressed himself by drawing pictures and talking about his life in the facility. He constantly asked his mother when he would be coming home, which led to great feelings of guilt on Eliza's part. He would soon be off on other subjects. His testing at the Manhattan Children's Psychiatric Center indicated that he was impulsive, with little planning or organizational ability and no ability for self-correction. Adam worked best in a very structured environment. Eliza had a difficult time setting up such structure in his life. We began by establishing some structure within our time together. I taught Eliza how to set boundaries in a nonjudgmental way. Early objectives were simple—having Eliza encourage Adam to sit still for a short time, and gradually lengthening the time requested. Eliza was coached to give Adam praise for the work he was able to do. We worked on Eliza's not being judgmental when he was unable to reach his objectives.

Adam could respond well to limit-setting, but he was so active that constant vigilance and active intervention were required. Given Eliza's own depression, she often found herself exhausted after a session with Adam. Eventually, we worked toward setting up a daytime visit at home, followed later by an overnight visit. We designed a schedule that would be posted on the refrigerator at home, detailing the structure for Adam's visit. Every hour of the visit was accounted for in our plan.

Throughout the process, Eliza expressed a great deal of concern about her son. Her greatest worry was that he would "turn out bad" and get himself killed on the streets. She took an active role in advocating for his care. She was able to execute plans that were put into place within our sessions. In one session, Adam was constantly shaking and seemed subdued compared with prior sessions. Eliza immediately demanded that he be taken off whatever medications he was taking. Eliza became disillusioned with the care he was receiving, particularly regarding his educational needs. She took the initiative to request help from a lawyer to protect Adam's rights. In conjunction with a colleague from the local neighborhood law center, Eliza and I successfully negotiated the placement of Adam in a specialized rehabilitation facility out of state. This ended the family therapy sessions for a period of 3½ years.

With the specialized intervention Adam was receiving, he made great gains in his rehabilitation. Adam was completing self-care tasks with a minimum of verbal cues. He was also improving his verbal problem-solving skills. His functional reading skills were not up to grade level but were improving. Eliza made regular trips to see him at the facility. He again began to pressure her about coming home. His mother had likewise progressed in her individual therapy.

Once Adam was in a productive setting for his rehabilitation, Eliza was able to work on hers. She became an active member of a therapy group. She took on a series of volunteer jobs with increasing responsibilities. Her affect improved and she became more outgoing. She began to think about the ways in which she could make productive contributions to the organized community of people with disabilities. She began attending community meetings as an advocate for homeless people with disabilities.

Adam continued to press Eliza to bring him home. Eliza felt guilty about Adam's being away for so long. She had ambivalent feelings about her ability to set limits with him. With the strides they had both made, Adam's therapist and I began to make plans for home visitations that would start with a weekend at home and eventually lead up to a couple of weeks at home, in preparation for the time when Adam might be returned to Eliza. It was still determined that Adam needed to be in a structured atmosphere. The major remaining question was whether Eliza and Adam could work together to create that atmosphere at home.

As we were beginning to put our transition plan in place, the City of New York decided that it no longer wanted to continue its contract with the rehabilitation facility that Adam was in. With very little notice, Adam was transferred to a school in Pennsylvania. Eliza was very upset about the transfer because it had been done without her consent. She immediately requested that he be brought home. I began working with a case manager from the child protection agency that had been responsible for Adam's placements. The major problem we faced was a catch-22 within the system. In the past, Eliza had received Aid to Dependent Children (AFDC) for Adam's care. On the basis of his placement, the City of New York had applied for Supplemental Security Income (SSI) for Adam, thus no longer making him eligible for AFDC. The case manager could not figure out how to transfer Adam's SSI from the City of New York to his mother. As a result, Adam was sent home with no means for his support. By this time, Adam was a teenager with a voracious appetite and the need for new clothes. Eliza was left for a period of 3 months with only her own SSI check for $520 a month to support both of them.

As soon as Adam returned home, we began to have family sessions again. Adam was more relaxed than he had been before, but he had a tendency to be taciturn within our sessions. Adam did not understand the financial dilemma his mother was in. His main interest was in getting new clothes so he could fit in with his old friends from the neighborhood. Eliza was very anxious about her situation. Her anxiety surfaced in the kind of statements she made to Adam. The goal of our initial sessions was to address the very real problem of not having money to make ends meet while working with both Eliza and Adam to develop coping skills to see their way through the crisis.

In the midst of the crisis, Eliza's diabetes went out of control, and she lost her kidney functions. Starting dialysis was a major blow to Eliza at a time when she was having trouble coping with the familial and fiscal changes in her life. We were finally able to get Adam's SSI transferred to his mother, but the damage was done. Given the fact that stress is a major factor in the control of diabetes, the changes Eliza was forced to endure proved to be too much for her. Six months after she started dialysis, she died in her sleep one Saturday night. During that

6-month period, her declining health caused her to miss many of her therapy sessions. I could see a spiral of declining physical health interacting with a concomitant decline in mental health.

After Eliza's death, Eliza's brother appeared to take care of his nephew. He seemed to put more energy into gaining custody of Eliza's old apartment than Eliza's son, Adam. Adam ended up splitting his time between living with his older brother and living with his uncle. I offered to help the family with the issues of grieving and adjusting to this new family configuration, but there was no interest forthcoming. The last word I had from the family was that Adam's uncle was sending him back to the school in Pennsylvania that his mother had resisted him attending.

~

With the present emphasis on cutting back on social services, I see the possibility for many other situations similar to Eliza's to arise. Too often policies are redesigned without considering the negative impact on the lives of the people who had been better served by earlier policies. Because of this tendency, being a therapist for people with disabilities often requires the additional role of becoming their advocate. A therapist cannot address issues of quality of life and familial communication if the family's ability to have food and shelter is called into question. Accordingly, it is not only helpful, but often necessary to establish a network of support with city, state, and private agencies. But there is no guarantee that, once services are in place, they will remain intact throughout the therapy process. In this era of budget-cutting, a therapist can safely assume that this is an area of concern that will have to be revisited regularly.

It can be very seductive for the therapist to substitute one system of family dependence for another in which the therapist becomes advocate and caregiver. Our critical task is to balance our roles as therapists and advocates in such a way that individuals with disabilities and their families have the support they need for negotiating the system while developing the skills they need to advocate for themselves. As the system of care is transformed, this will require reeducation for empowerment for both the individuals and families we serve as well as for ourselves.

9

Gilbert

Lost in Time

Mary Ann Blotzer

Gilbert keeps searching for his father. He looks for him in the torn-off calendar pages that he pulls from trash cans. "When is my father coming back from dead?" he plaintively asks me. In his late forties, with both autism and mental retardation, Gilbert struggles to make sense of a world that he lacks the mental structures to comprehend.

Mental retardation and autism have profound consequences upon one's ability to understand and cope with life. It is not simply that being slower or different makes life harder; rather the defining characteristics of these disabilities can create nearly insurmountable obstacles to understanding one's experiences and coping effectively with life. Autism is characterized by disturbances of language, and in the ability to relate to others, and sometimes disturbances in sensory perception and integration. Persons with autism can be overly reactive to certain forms of sensory stimulation and may have great difficulty organizing the material that comes through their senses. The sound of a vacuum cleaner, for example, can be excruciatingly painful. While under the barrage of this sound, the person with autism may be unable to focus upon anything else other than trying to endure what for him is sensory torture. When overly stimulated in this way, the individual with autism may seem to be "in his own world"—a world that is inpenetrable to others.

Sensory integration can also be severely impaired with autism. The ability that most individuals take for granted—the ability to integrate sensory data from one sense or location with that from another—is profoundly lacking. Donna Williams, an Australian who has published two books about her experience of autism, refers to her lack of "any connected inner body sense" (1994, p. 217) and describes her lack of sensory integration for even the same sense—in this case, touch: "If I touched my leg I would feel it on my hand or leg but not both at the same time. My perception of a whole body was in bits. I was an arm or a leg or a nose" (p. 232). Like the newborn with undeveloped integrative capacities who must close her eyes to suck at the breast, but cannot simultaneously gaze at her mother and suck (Alvarez, 1992), the individual with autism may lack the ability to synthesize sensory data into a unified, coherent system. This leads to both a fragmented sense of the world and even of self. Compounding these difficulties are the language difficulties. Donna Williams eloquently describes her moments of receptive aphasia as going "meaning deaf": she hears words, but they are unconnected to meaning. Some individuals with autism appear to experience central aphasia, "an impaired capacity to use language for thinking, for 'talking to oneself'" (Seifert, 1990, p. 51). Thus, the language difficulties inherent in autism serve to alienate the person with autism from even his own experience and complicate the development of a sense of self. And when self is confused, how can self meet other?

It is no wonder that persons with autism are seldom thought of as candidates for psychotherapy. The technical obstacles are enormous. Persons with autism perceive and organize their experiences differently, and their difficulties with language mean that it is very hard for them to tell us directly about their experience. Therapists faced with such clients must first develop some framework for understanding how persons with autism perceive, encode, and communicate their experiences.

To enter into the psychotherapeutic relationship with someone with autism is to risk feeling disoriented, lost, confused, and inadequate. But we must first understand their world if we are to invite them to join ours. And we must first determine where they are lost, before we can bring them to safety. And we must first be willing to bear their chaos, before we can help them to order it.

This chapter describes the therapeutic journey of one patient, Gilbert, who struggles with the limitations of both autism and mental retardation. It discusses major themes in therapy and also strategies devised to help Gilbert through the therapeutic process—or, said another way, strategies to help the therapist reach through to the patient past the obstacles that disabilities present.

Most therapy patients have the capacity to organize their experience into a narrative flow. Indeed, some professionals would contend that this ability is essential if one is to benefit from therapy. We take this ability and the sense and order that it brings to our lives for granted. But what if one lacks this synthetic ability to pull the strands of one's experience together? Then life may feel unbearably chaotic and unpredictable. Gilbert largely lives in a world of perception without integration and of time without history. Because it is so difficult for Gilbert to make sense and order out of what feel like disparate strands of experience, he has developed certain strategies that provide him with a sense of order and control. Over time as these strategies have comforted him, they have become calcified into the static quality of rituals. Although these rituals comfort him, they impede him from further growth. They become autistic comforts that serve to both soothe and further isolate him.

Events that inherently signal change—beginnings and endings, stoppings and startings, and comings and goings—frighten Gilbert. I have come to understand this as his difficulty organizing and holding onto the chunks of his experience and then weaving these discrete chunks into a whole that constitutes the sense of a unified life. Because of the compartmentalized quality of Gilbert's experience (a quality largely caused by the sensory difficulties associated with his autism), he lacks a sense of personal continuity and the continuity of experience. This lack is evidenced by Gilbert's inability to relate a narrative. Even very young children can report, "I went here. And then this happened. Next I did this." But at most, Gilbert will make a simple statement such as, "I went to the picnic, Mary Ann." He never adds, "I went to the picnic and then it rained, so we went home." Gilbert typically speaks in one of two ways: simple declarative sentences or hypothetical questions. Gilbert's hypotheticals are always concerned with time, as shown in his question, "What would happen if tomorrow were Tuesday?" While one might think that these hypothetical questions reflect greater abstract abilities, the fact that these are always the same form of question about time indicates otherwise. Later I will share my thinking on the function of time in Gilbert's personal universe.

Because of Gilbert's deficient sense of continuity, I wonder whether he alternately fears falling into personal oblivion or into chaos. When traveling on the London subway, the conductor, a disembodied voice over a loudspeaker, repeatedly intones, "Mind the gap," as the train stops at stations where there is a large space between the train doors and the platform. With Gilbert, I am always conscious of the gap in his experience. Gilbert could easily fall through the cracks.

~

Related to his difficulty with narrative flow is his need to manage temporal transitions and make concrete that which is abstract. Gilbert employs rigid and predictable strategies to manage the countless moments each day that signal change and to attempt to solidify his experiences so that they become more real and permanent. As his therapist, it is my job to support his efforts for control, predictability, and permanence. In addition, I must bring his rituals into mindful awareness. My hope is that talking with him about what he is trying to achieve will enable him to make subtle transformations.

Gilbert's notions of place and time fuel his rituals. Because of the strong concrete quality to his thinking, his internal representations of place and time are equally concrete. For example, Gilbert asks me, "When will my father be back from dead?" "Will you be in your office on Saturday, Mary Ann?" "Where do you live, Mary Ann?" To Gilbert, being dead is a place. And in order to hold onto a sense of me, he needs to place me. Where am I when I'm not with him? How can he be certain of my continued existence? By locating me in space (e.g., in my office on Saturday or at my home on Mondays), Gilbert helps himself to maintain a mental sense of me.

I consider how Gilbert thinks and conduct the therapy with as much awareness of this as I am capable of. But I do not always understand how he thinks. I am constantly generating hypotheses and testing them out. Sometimes I make what feel like hopeless stabs in the dark. At times, Gilbert lets me know that I have bridged the gap. Being with Gilbert is sometimes disorienting to me as I attempt to understand the world as he sees it. I must then take abstract notions, distill them to the concrete, and then share these with Gilbert. The process makes me feel like a translator at the United Nations. When, early in his therapy, Gilbert would ask me, "When will my father come back from dead?" I viewed this as Gilbert's difficulty making sense of death due to his concreteness. I would respond equally concretely as follows: "People don't come back from being dead." On some level Gilbert thought of being dead as a place, and it made sense for me to use this sense of death as a place in my responses to him. Later in the therapy, I would bridge more gaps between the concrete and the abstract. I frequently wonder how much therapy can help Gilbert to expand how he thinks. Are his mental structures relatively immutable, or can he develop an expanded capacity for organizing and processing his experiences?

To this end, I use Gilbert's need to firmly fix me in a location as a bridge to *thinking about thinking about me*. I begin with the concrete, and then move a step toward the mental representation. For example, when Gilbert would ask me, "Will you be in your office on Saturday?" I sensed that this was his way of thinking about me and of wondering where I was when I was not with him. He needed a better fix on my existence. So I would talk about the times and places when I was with him and about the other times and places: "You see me here in my office on Mondays, but other times I'm at my home or out doing things. On Sundays, you can *remind yourself* that you will see me on Mondays."

~

We take for granted our ability to hold onto a mental image of another person or thing. This ability is basic for *thinking about* the other. When we miss someone we can comfort ourselves by evoking a mental image of the person we miss. Our inner lives are richly populated with these images of the important figures in our lives and with our emotional associations to them. This capacity, while not wholly lacking in Gilbert, is significantly impaired. He needs help in other ways to develop these images, to think about them, and to hold onto them to use both to comfort himself and as tools for thinking about the others. His strategies for doing so are what can make him seem so odd. For example, one of his strategies is to overly orient people in space and in time. Witness his oft-repeated line of questioning to me, "Will you be in your office tomorrow, Mary Ann? Where do you live?" These are not idle, meaningless questions. They are rich in the depth of meaning they convey about the strategies Gilbert uses to hold onto an inner sense of people and about his worries. Gilbert's biggest fear is that people will disappear; particularly his mother, and me, his other mother-object. His sudden loss of his father has much to do with this fear.

Gilbert's mother, with whom he lived, referred him to me within a few months of his father's death. His father had died after a brief and sudden hospitalization. Totally unprepared for this, in shock, and having difficulty comprehending the loss and ordering it into his experience in a meaningful fashion, Gilbert deteriorated rapidly into a withdrawn, disorganized, nearly psychotic state. Activities that he had previously completed with ease, such as his household chores or work routines, were only possible with massive amounts of support and guidance. Although he was fortunate to be receiving services from a vocational agency, he was having such difficulty getting through the day that his job was in serious jeopardy. He simply could not maintain his focus long enough to sustain any but the most basic of activities. He was alternately disorganized and giggly or aggressive. Set adrift by grief, he was unable to meaningfully focus his attention or organize his activity.

"Mary Ann, when will my father be back from dead?" This was Gilbert's mournful, oft-repeated cry to me throughout the first year of his therapy. Like most initial statements from patients in therapy, it was emblematic of his larger difficulties. It reflected both his difficulty understanding death, and his deep desire to have the depth of his grief understood by another human being. Gilbert's autism and mental retardation leave him with an impaired capacity to fully comprehend much of what happens to him. At the same time, Gilbert deeply craves understanding. My job as his therapist has been to work deeply to understand him, and just as deeply to find a way of communicating my understanding back to him. Given the idiosyncracies of communication that are the hallmark of autism, this task has been extremely challenging.

My work with Gilbert and with other persons who have autism has convinced me that conventional notions about the desires of persons with autism are mistaken. Contrary to the belief that individuals with autism crave their aloofness from others, preferring things to people, my clinical experience has convinced me that they crave connection to others and the sense of being deeply understood. But their desire for closeness and understanding must be met in a way that is tolerable to them. The first person account of Donna Williams (Williams, 1994), a woman with autism, supports this view.

Perhaps Gilbert's greatest strength is his drive to be understood. But because of his autism, he expresses this in ways that seem bizarre and devoid of meaning. To the uninitiated, his questions seem silly; truly, they do set him apart. In fact, his seemingly bizarre line of questions prompted his vocational staff to modify his behavioral program. A new goal was added: Gilbert was to have "interesting conversations." Whenever Gilbert would repeat himself or ask when his dad would be back "from dead," his job coach, Lucy, would respond, "Have interesting conversations, Gilbert." Gilbert, ever eager to please, would reply, "I'll have interesting conversations. Okay, Lucy?" while mimicking a smile that seemed more a grimace. Gilbert frantically craves acceptance from others and hence tries to figure out what is expected of him and to comply so as to be accepted. But given his disabilities, it is often difficult for him to discern just what is expected from him. The directive, "have interesting conversations," provided no useful information as to what constituted an "interesting conversation." About all that he took from it was that it was a cue to stop talking about whatever he was talking about at the time. Furthermore, I suspect that Gilbert often goes "meaning deaf." Words are nothing but meaningless sounds to him because he has temporarily lost the ability to decode these sounds. When this occurs, he uses his tried and true strategy for trying to placate people: He mimics whatever the person has just said. This provides the illusion that he has understood them. Hence, he replied to Lucy, "I'll have interesting conversations. Okay,

Lucy?" The "Okay, Lucy?" was said in the tone of a child who wants reassurance that the adult is not angry with him.

Over time, as I have learned Gilbert's language, the quality of his relatedness has improved. We were able to have meaningful exchanges that lasted longer. Again, I have seen this phenomenon in other persons with autism. Only after I join them in their world, using their language, can I gradually bring them to join more of the world that those of us unaffected by autism inhabit and to speak in a more direct fashion. Now, after seeing Gilbert for many years, I can more quickly bridge the gap between the oddness of what he is saying and the real issue he wants to talk about. When he asks me, "Why won't my father be there [at a holiday dinner]?" I can respond, "Perhaps you want to say how much you miss your father and how hard it is to get used to his being gone." It is difficult to adequately describe the shift that occurs when my "translation" hits the mark. But there is an almost palpable softening and relaxing in the room. Sometimes Gilbert will become quiet and say, "Yeah." The effect is that he seems to have absorbed my interpretation and experienced it in a meaningful way. At other times he will follow up with more direct questions on the same theme. But whether he responds with a connected quietness that expresses a settling in or by talking more about the issue, there is a very real sense of connection between us.

This quality is vastly different from the quality that permeates my office when I miss the mark. At these times there's a sense of us talking past one another. I spend a lot of time feeling lost, stupid, and inadequate when I see persons with autism. Some of this is because I am the object into which they project their intolerable feelings of being lost, stupid, and inadequate. But to be honest, it is also because I am often unsure of my bearings. My understanding of what is transpiring in the interview feels incomplete and I feel quite inadequate to the task of understanding this person and of bridging the gap between his experience and that of the outer world. As painful as this is, it is sometimes a good thing. Being able to bear this sense of uncertainty and inadequacy and to work through it is what maintains the connection between my patient and myself. After all, I suspect that Gilbert spends most of his life feeling uncertain and inadequate. Our shared experience of this is an unconscious communication that is central to our work.

~

Gilbert went through a period of heightened obsession with calendars. He would become agitated when he saw cast-off calendar pages in trash cans. He would frantically insist on retrieving them. The end of each month was a time of heightened turmoil for him. About this same time, he asked me if his father would still have birthdays and if the year was 1985 (the year before his father died). I suggested that perhaps he wanted to go back in time to find his father. This seemed to calm him, and he asked more questions about the time of his father's life. Concretely, I talked about the months and years during which his father had been alive. Then I talked about the months that had passed since his death. Next I talked about the months and years in the future, during which Gilbert's father would remain dead. Gilbert seemed to respond to this concrete grounding of past, present, and future, and for several sessions we repeated the process. This line of conversation, which Gilbert insisted on going over for many weeks, is now far in the past. It no longer speaks to his present circumstances. Now what Gilbert seems to most want from me is empathy. Periodically he brings up his father, and I generally interpret this as his way of wanting me to know how much he misses his father and of wanting to hold onto his memory. This seems to satisfy Gilbert and he moves on. But if I had attempted this months before, before I had made the effort to learn Gilbert's way of speaking, it would not have been meaningful to Gilbert. I think he would have perceived it as just one more unattuned person talking at him.

Gilbert's disability seems to have also affected his grounding in time, another problem that makes it difficult for him to order his experience. Much like young children who "can't wait" for events that they eagerly anticipate, Gilbert literally "can't wait" for events that are in the near future. Most of us take for granted the adaptive advantages that an adult sense of time provides. It enables us to manage our anxiety, to anticipate future events, and to generally feel securely anchored. We know that the passage of 3 days feels different from the passage of 1 day and that 3 weeks is three times longer than 1 week. This linear sense of time enables us to pace ourselves and to plan accordingly. We measure days in equal intervals. Gilbert, in contrast, experiences time differently. His level of anticipation for an event that is to happen in 3 days is nearly the same as that for an event that is to happen in 1 hour.

Because Gilbert's inner life is chaotic and because he lacks the necessary internal mental structures for understanding and ordering outside experience, he craves rigid predictability and tries to create it where it does not exist. Thus, if someone visits him on a Saturday, he wants to insist that that person will come every Saturday. And upon being told that this will not happen, he becomes very confused and disturbed, which leads him to engage in another line of perseverative questioning. I suspect that being Gilbert is deeply exhausting; there is so much for him to try to keep track of.

Gilbert is still fascinated by calendars—a fascination fueled by his drive to master the anxiety he experiences at the gap between his subjective experience of time and real time. To the uninitiated, Gilbert's questions about time can appear bizarre or comical. For example, after his birthday has fallen on a Tuesday, he might ask me, "Mary Ann, what would happen if next Tuesday were my birthday?" He becomes anxious by the closing of a month and is apt to ask, "Mary Ann, what if June had 31 days?" I take these questions seriously but not literally. They represent his attempts to better understand his experience.

Talking with Gilbert, as is the case with many patients who have autism, is a strange combination of the concrete and the metaphorical. Autism is characterized by the idiosyncratic use of language. Gilbert's disability makes it nearly impossible for him to communicate his concerns in a straightforward fashion. Many of Gilbert's comments would seem utterly meaningless if taken at face value, but they are his best attempt at saying what is on his mind. The responsibility falls on me and Gilbert's caregivers to translate his comments into understandable language and to then feed this back to him. Although Gilbert's thinking is extraordinarily concrete, I often must think metaphorically and associationally if I am to understand him. Most individuals have a more linear style of conversing. They remain on the same topic and the back and forth exchange flows logically and smoothly. But Gilbert does not operate under the same system of logic. How can he when his sense of time and other perceptions create a different universe? Gilbert often responds by associating to something that I have said. Following the thread of these associations is typically very productive. In this way Gilbert communicates his concerns and I can better understand him. Our conversations have their own logic: a logic based on his way of thinking.

A mother says to her preschool-age child, "I love you more than you can imagine." It's a statement that acknowledges the gap between the sense of the mother and the limits of the imagination of the child. Yet it also implies that the child can acknowledge the gap between her awareness and something greater than her awareness—her mother's love for her.

After I had been seeing Gilbert for a few years and he had recovered to his previous level of functioning, his married brother who had spent untold amounts of time with him announced that he was being transferred out of the country. Frank, the brother, was remarkably empathetic and had a wonderful sense of Gilbert. He could almost always understand what Gilbert was saying and communicate this understanding back to Gilbert.

Frank's departure was planned, and Gilbert and I began talking about it 2 months in advance. Unlike his father's death, we could anticipate this loss (think about it happening in the near future) and talk about it. Although Gilbert had some sense that Frank was leaving, it took the passage of time for the reality to sink in. Gilbert used to spend the last weekend of every month at Frank's house. Three weeks after Frank's move, when the last weekend of the month had come and gone, the reality of Frank's departure began to sink in. At that time Gilbert became increasingly tearful and agitated. When he arrived in my office that week he could barely contain himself. He was disruptive in the waiting room and was unable to tolerate sitting by himself when his mother went in to talk with me. Watching Gilbert, who was distraught, tearful, and disorganized, was painful. All he could do was to cry, pace aimlessly, blow his nose into his hand, and then smear his face with nasal mucus. I remember feeling terribly inadequate; how could I help this man who was hurting so deeply and who was becoming disorganized by his grief? In what felt like a feeble attempt to help, I said that perhaps he was showing me how undone he was by his sadness. This seemed to settle him a bit and I went on to talk about missing Frank. Gilbert then asked, "When will my father be back from dead?" and I wondered aloud if he felt that he had lost Frank in this final way too. All that I could do was bear witness to Gilbert's pain and sadness and offer empathetic comments. Intermittently, Gilbert would get up from his chair to come hug me or to pat my hair. He was consoling himself by touching me and I commented on this.

The following week Gilbert had shifted. No longer distraught and agitated, he seemed to have retreated into a depressive position. As soon as he walked into my office, he curled up in the chair as though to go to sleep, picking up the throw pillow on a chair and cradling it in his arms. He spent most of the session this way, saying little, but appearing to be comforted by the opportunity to curl up in the chair hugging the pillow. I wondered aloud whether he was worn out by his grief and becoming resigned to Frank's move overseas. Gilbert simply replied, "I'm upset."

Gilbert's depressive withdrawal felt appropriate to me. He did not feel aloof in an autistic sense, but simply sad and quiet as anyone would be as the reality of a loss sinks in. Frank's departure brought a reprise of Gilbert's grief for his father. And as often is the case when therapy is effective, the issue can be worked through at a deeper level and resolved more readily. So it was for Gilbert. I think that my ability to witness and share his sadness, to provide support through his grief, and to comment empathically enabled him to better manage his feelings.

When talking to a colleague about this work, we both shared our questions regarding the adequacy and accuracy of our interpretations. Many of our patients with autism say little or talk in a bizarre fashion. We turn ourselves inside out attempting to understand their meaning, and then again to communicate our understanding back to them. Each of us has ways of assessing whether our comments resonate with our patients or miss the mark. Sometimes the result is subtle—a quieting in a patient who is usually agitated. But sometimes our patients do let us know when they have felt understood or misunderstood by us. At times our interpretations stimulate healing, but perhaps the real curative factor in therapy is that our patients know that we are desperately trying to understand them and to make sense of their communications.

I think of Gilbert especially in this regard. To the untrained observer, most of what Gilbert says seems repetitive or bizarre. Comments such as, "When is my father coming back from dead?" when Gilbert knows that death is forever, or "Mary Ann, will I see you next Wednesday?" when we've spent the past half hour discussing the fact that I will be on vacation the next week, can seem meaningless, just the odd rantings of an odd person. But instead I take my best stab at expressing what Gilbert might want to express and offer this back to him to see if he can make use of it. Perhaps, "When is my father coming back from dead?" means "I still miss my father very much. It's hard to accept his death. I need you to know this." Perhaps when he says, "Mary Ann, will I see you next Monday?" what he really wants to say is, "I don't like it when you go on vacation. I miss coming here, and I always worry when people go away. I like knowing where people are at all times." I certainly do not always bat a thousand when I offer my interpretations to Gilbert, but perhaps what is most important is that Gilbert knows that I take him seriously, even when I don't understand him. The other important dimension to this process is that the continual give and take keeps us engaged in a relationship. If I were to simply dismiss his comments as bizarre, our relationship would be very superficial.

My best description of this process is that I take the patient seriously, but not literally. No matter how odd the remark sounds, I try to find in it the keys to understanding what the person is really trying to communicate. I then reflect these possibilities back to the person, seeking his or her corrective feedback. Although accurate interpretations can clearly have a healing, transformative effect, the sustained effort to maintain connection and to understand can also be a curative factor. Connection and understanding are also communicated nonverbally. Persons with autism are easily overwhelmed by sensory stimulation, including proximity to another person. I work hard to avoid overwhelming Gilbert by my voice, my movements, even my breathing and the directness of my gaze.

When thinking about Gilbert I find it useful to generate hypotheses about his internal mental processes. What structures does he have for digesting, organizing, holding, and mentally manipulating his experiences? How rudimentary or developed are these capacities? Which seem more likely to develop with focused interventions, and which are more productively thought of as enduring deficits? Can he be assisted with what I call "prosthetic mental structures?" The use of a prosthetic mental structure can best be illustrated by another patient with autism, Alma.

Alma was described by her residential staff as "obsessed with death." She would talk endlessly about celebrities who had died. But it was not a macabre fascination with death that fueled her remarks. Her comments on death were part of her broader focus upon change, transformation, and loss. For example, when what had once been a fast food restaurant changed hands and became a bowling alley, Alma wanted to know what happened to the hamburgers that had been there. A friend of mine, the mother of a 2-year-old, related an exchange with her daughter that reflected the difficulties that ensue when immature cognitive structures attempt to process loss and transformation. The child's father had recently shaved off his mustache, and the family had a neighbor, Ben, who had a mustache. Seeking to understand this, the child had the following dialogue with her mother.

> Child: "Mommy, Daddy shaved off his mustache, right?"
> Mother: "Yes."
> Child: "Where did it go? I bet he gave it to Ben."

Like the child in this example, Alma lacked adequate mental processes and structures to mentally metabolize the many transformations inherent in life, whether it is the cancellation of a favorite television show, the changed purpose of a commercial building, or the many comings and goings of people, whether temporary (vacations, shift changes, moves) or permanent (death). While there was an emotional valence to her preoccupation with death and transformation, her lack of adequate conceptual structures also contributed to her "obsession."

Sometimes what we provide to our patients is a prosthetic mental structure—not the real thing, not something that is truly part of them, but something they can use to perform certain functions. When Alma would bring up the names of persons she knew who had died, her mother would respond, "You're remembering (name)." Alma was able to latch onto this and use it, much like a prosthetic limb. She didn't use it as fluently as she would if it were truly hers, but it helped her. To say, "You're remembering (name)" seemed to move her a step toward greater integration. It also provided an opening to talk more about remembering and missing, mental processes intimately tied to the capacity for relatedness.

This intersection of cognitive processes (e.g., the cognitive ability to understand loss, change, transformation) and the emotional valence attached to these issues are important to consider when treating persons with autism or related difficulties. Both elements must be addressed. Gilbert has cognitive difficulties understanding death, as well as feelings surrounding his father's death. These interact, and interventions must be designed with both elements in mind.

~

Inconclusive Thoughts. Despite our best attempts to understand another human being, we can never precisely know how another feels. When we ache for our child who is sick, it is not our child's pain that we feel, but an imagined facsimile that is deeply rooted in our own unique experience. Our imaginative capacity is all that we have in our efforts to bridge the gap that separates us. We are each a self inside a skin. And it is our own self that we draw on when attempting to understand another. We go about it egocentrically, thinking that others are like us. But what if the self inside that other skin perceives and organizes his experience in a completely different style? And what if that different perceptual style makes it hard to even develop a coherent sense of self? Such is the case when persons without autism attempt to relate to persons with autism. I had to begin my work with Gilbert by throwing out my own experience. My own experience was no guide to understanding him.

I agree with Anne Alvarez of the Tavistock Clinic who wrote, "Such patients can be helped by psychoanalytic methods, but the treatment is long, arduous, and almost always places considerable strain on the therapist. *Yet there is growing consensus that this strain and burden is in some way central to the treatment*" (1992, p. ix; italics added). The confusion and disorientation that I have felt in working with Gilbert mirror his state of mind, and, as such, my experience of this is essential if he is to be helped by our encounter.

I believe that it is this reluctance to tolerate uncertainty, including uncertainties about one's adequacies as a therapist, that leads to the dismissal of entire groups of people as candidates for therapy. Persons with autism are often treated as though autism was a collection of behavioral oddities rather than "a system of making sense of things" (Williams, 1994, p. 199). As a system, it severely taxes both the individual with autism and those who try to relate to him or her. My work with Gilbert has been guided by my belief that I must first understand how he experiences his world before I can even attempt to help him to share the world that persons without autism experience. This work is both intellectually and emotionally taxing. It requires that I generate hypotheses about his perceptions and representations and then test these out. Truly, it requires a deep capacity to sit with uncertainty.

REFERENCES

Alvarez, A. (1992). *Live company: Psychoanalytic psychotherapy with autistic, borderline, deprived and abused children*. London: Routledge.
Seifert, C. (1990). *Theories of autism*. Lanham, MD: University Park Press.
Williams, D. (1994). *Somebody somewhere*. New York: Times Books.

10

Amy

A Young Woman Chooses to Be Mute

Jean Finkelstein Ratner

Amy was 20 years old when she became electively mute. She spoke only rarely. When she did speak, it was about religious or science fiction characters or she spoke in a private language that no one but she could understand. The referral for therapy came to me from a colleague who had seen Amy in individual, activity-oriented therapy for 2 years without significant change.

The case was a very puzzling and troubling one. I knew from Amy's prior therapist that Amy was the youngest of 10 children in a very loving, active, and devout family. Family members all spent a great deal of time with Amy. As a child and young adolescent, she had been quiet but responded warmly to affection. She had participated actively in the life of the family. She did various chores, said grace at meals, and read cards aloud at family celebrations. Her verbal skills were remarkably strong, given her retardation. In addition to her work at a sheltered workshop, she had been busy with various church and community activities. She enjoyed sports, such as shooting baskets with a brother, and was in the Special Olympics several times.

At age 20, Amy withdrew gradually but markedly from everyone and everything she had seemed to enjoy so much before. She no longer would initiate any conversation and did not call family members by name. If she addressed her mother at all, on the rare occasion when she spoke, she mysteriously chose "Pam" as a name to call her. Amy acknowledged that she had a private language. Questions to her were met with silence. Her thoughts, which she almost always kept to herself, centered around spiritual matters and science fiction. Both auditory and visual hallucinations appeared to be present when she mumbled to St. John, to Yahweh (God), or to characters from Star Trek. An imaginary, male friend was occasionally mentioned. Amy no longer said grace at meals nor would she read out loud. Family activities were no longer a source of pleasure, and her prior participation gave way to detachment. If the others swam in the pool, she remained sitting on the edge. If they walked, she fell behind. Eye contact was rare and fleeting when it did occur. Everything was done more slowly at home and at work. Even her handwriting deteriorated from neat, legible printing to a loose, illegible scrawl.

Her parents were deeply concerned when they brought her to our mental health center, which is known in the community for its psychotherapy for adults with developmental disabilities. After a careful evaluation, our team thought that Amy's withdrawal had been precipitated by two successive losses of siblings, both of whom had married and moved out from the family home within 2 years of each other. A tremendous void was left in Amy's life. Depression and silence may have been the result of overwhelming grief.

My colleague, who had used activity therapy with Amy, was an unusually warm and nurturing therapist. She had attempted in many ways to build an alliance with this distant, withdrawn young woman. In Amy's drawings, the therapist saw her repeatedly drawing circles which she darkened in with more circles. When she drew figures, Amy identified them as "Vampire" and "Jack the Ripper." She spoke of Yahweh (God), and, if she spoke of herself, it was not using the pronoun "I" but in the distancing third person. The therapist spoke of some of the underlying issues and feelings that she saw in Amy's drawings: "feeling lost" and anger. After 2 years of activity therapy, Amy showed a bit more connectedness to the therapist and her face showed more animated expression, but she remained largely detached and mute. To rule out Alzheimer's disease, which can occur in young adults with Down syndrome, a referral was made to an inpatient research program. Alzheimer's disease was ruled out.

Amy's therapist asked our team to reconsider the initial treatment plan. We had learned over the years that our initial plan for any patient with significant developmental disabilities was not always the plan that would be ultimately effective. We find that when individual therapy fails, we may add or shift entirely to group therapy. There have been other times when we have begun with group therapy, but changed to individual therapy. In Amy's case at this point, the team thought it would be worth a try to bring Amy into a group that I was co-leading. Amy would be able to hear from peers in the group about significant losses in their lives that came up frequently in their families, group homes, and worksites.

An appointment was set up for me to meet Amy. Her mother and therapist would be there. When I entered the room, I was immediately struck by how much this petite young woman looked like a girl of 13 or 14 rather than her 24 years. She was perched stiffly on the front of her chair with a worried expression, head cocked a bit to one side, eyes darting but not staying with either her mother or the therapist she had worked with for 2 years. As she lifted her arms behind her head and waved her fingers, my thoughts immediately went to the stereotypical movements of autism, but I knew that Amy had related too nicely to others during childhood and adulthood for that diagnosis to be correct. It would not be for another year that I would hear that work was being done at the National Institute of Mental Health (NIMH) with patients with Asperger's disorder, a newly recognized diagnosis for higher-level patients who showed some autistic features. Perhaps Amy could be reevaluated at the NIMH sometime in the future when she could better withstand another evaluation. For now, her diagnosis would remain Major Depression.

I had fully expected Amy to come into my therapy group, but sitting now in the room with her, feeling the severity of her detachment and sensing her terror, I realized she would be overwhelmed by our noisy group. It seemed wiser to see her individually for however long it would take to forge the beginning of an alliance.

~

My role as a therapist becomes an unusually active one when I work with a client who is severely withdrawn. I often request that a family member or house counselor come in weekly to meet with the client and me either immediately before or after the individual session. In these conjoint sessions, I can obtain detailed information about the patient's life. This may include material about the distant past, events of the prior week, or events expected in the weeks to come. I ask for very detailed information, exacting descriptions of people, events, places, and how the client appeared to react or feel at the time. These images obtained from the significant other person in the conjoint session can often arouse the attention of the most withdrawn client and elicit strong reactions. These reactions can engage the client with whatever reality must be faced.

In my thoughts about the use of details to engage Amy, I was drawing from remarkable lectures by the late Dr. Alvin Semrad, Professor of Psychiatry at Harvard Medical School, who was the preeminent teacher of graduate social work students as well as psychiatrists in the Boston community some 25 years before. He was known as a wise and caring physician who would leave jargon behind and use simple words to reach any patient, including the most resistant. He taught new therapists to investigate the details of a patient's experience, the aspects of life most important to him or her, in order to release repressed feelings. "The technique of therapy," said Semrad, "can be to go over and over the facts—to pick up the cues omitted from consideration at the time" (Rako & Mazer, 1980, p. 110). "Go after the specific details of the experience so you can help the patient recall what he has repressed in order to avoid" (p. 113). And with patients who seemed out of touch with reality, the depth of Semrad's empathic approach was clear: "You wonder if they ever did anything very interesting in their lives or whether it was all emptiness and failure . . . Well, you can bet your bottom dollar about one thing they did: once upon a time they loved somebody" (Rako & Mazer, 1980, p. 140).

In the conjoint session, I am actively engaged with the parent or counselor gathering information, but we are not talking as if the client were not there. While we speak, I face the client and try to make eye contact with him or her. I often restate to the client what I have just heard from the parent or counselor to emphasize its importance. As I repeat it, I translate it into a "you" statement to help the client feel connected to rather than removed from the events that have taken place. If the mother or father tells me about the details of another daughter's marriage, I next turn to the client and repeat the story saying, "Your sister got married. . . ." In this way, we establish a framework built on facts: the who, when, where, what, and why. From there we can begin to talk about a range of feelings people are likely to feel in such a situation: happy, excited, sad, disappointed, angry, frustrated. I stress to the parent or counselor the importance of speaking of his or her own feelings in the situation or a similar one as a way of role modeling the expression of appropriate feelings for our client. And so I might ask the parent at this point, "How did *you* feel about the wedding?"

In the case of a largely silent client who can easily feel overwhelmed or intimidated, I do not push if the client does not respond to my statements or will not answer questions. The client is allowed to remain silent. I may verbalize a hunch, such as, "The wedding was a time when everyone was excited. Maybe you were excited too, and maybe you were also sad because you knew your sister was moving to her own home after the wedding." The client usually does not respond verbally at this early stage, but there may be nonverbal reactions. Many times Amy slowly raised her arms to flutter her fingers rapidly behind her head. Or her eyes widened, and she looked frightened while she bounced forcefully in her chair. When this happened, I described the movements to Amy and wondered aloud if she was trying to tell me that she is very upset, perhaps frightened, about the topic at hand or another thought that may have come to her mind.

In this early period of therapy, in which the client is allowed to remain silent, there may be so much chaos inside the client that he or she is unable to think in terms of self, others, or relationships, let alone feelings. The therapist and significant other are doing most or all of the talking, trying to establish the facts of the client's world, the client's life story. Any therapist working with the silent client must be concerned about the possibility of "putting words into the client's mouth." The therapist faces a true dilemma: The therapist does not want the client to parrot ideas she has heard in therapy in some rote way. But neither does the therapist want to leave her floundering in silence with powerful feelings. Amy had already shown us in a prior nondirective therapy that she can remain immobilized indefinitely, drawing the classic circles of the autistic state. If a less directive therapy proves ineffective, perhaps a directive therapy even with all its risks may be tried to help the client move out of the "cold storage" phase (Tustin, 1986). The patient goes into "cold storage" for protection from internal chaos. In most therapies, the therapist loans his or her ego to a lesser or greater extent. In this highly directive therapy for the withdrawn, mute client, one loans ego substantially, but with caution.

When the therapist is this active, one must keep in mind that the patient may be agreeing out of a desire to be liked or because of the tendency autistic patients have to repeat the last word(s) heard. The presence of the family member or counselor who knows the client well is an important safeguard. Evaluating whether this client can say "no" or otherwise disagree with the therapist is very important. The therapist, when verbalizing hunches, would be wise to follow each hunch with a question that allows for disagreement: "Is that the way you felt, or was it different for you?" And when the autistic client is presented with options (such as "Were you frustrated, happy or sad?"), the order of positive and negative feelings should be presented in first one order and then in reverse order; however, in Amy's case, word order did not seem to influence her choice when presented with options.

Finally, the therapist needs to be aware of what is happening in the patient's life outside the therapy office. If the overall approach, however directive, resonates for the most part with the patient, we should begin to see some signs of change in the client. These changes may be subtle. If the significant other is a careful observer, important information about the client's behavior at home will be invaluable in gauging the client's reaction to the therapy. But if the overall approach reflects the therapist's bias and the therapist is putting words into the client's mouth, positive change is unlikely.

~

At the end of the first meeting when I was introduced to Amy, I invited her and her mother to my office so her mother could begin to tell me who the most important people have been in Amy's life. Amy's mother began telling me about each of her two adult children who had married and moved out, one soon after the other. She became tearful as she spoke of missing her infant granddaughter, Carolyn, whom she helped raise in her home from infancy. Carolyn's father, Amy's brother, had moved back home with Carolyn some years before, following a marital separation. One of the two marriages was the remarriage of this son who, of course, moved with his daughter and bride to their new home. For Amy's mother the marriages had been a source of joy, but it was quite difficult to see her granddaughter move out after so many years of having her in their home. The family had not talked about the sad side of these events which Amy's mother's tears expressed so poignantly. This loving and protective mother and grandmother had not wanted to detract from her granddaughter's joy at having two parents with whom she would live.

I explained to Amy and her mother that it would be extremely important for us to talk together about these changes in the family because they had happened to both of them, and it was clear there had been a lot of unexpressed sad feelings. Amy's mother picked up immediately on the idea that sharing her sadness now with Amy could help her silent daughter. Amy gave no visible reaction to my recommendation, but when she came to the clinic several days later to say goodbye to her prior therapist, I was told she stopped briefly outside my door.

With a mother so open to sharing grief that her daughter could not express, my thoughts were shifting away from group therapy to individual therapy with Amy and with both daughter and mother together. I asked to see Amy's mother one time alone before beginning. She agreed without hesitation. When she came in, she began by expressing surprise that children with developmental disabilities had such deep feelings. She shared with me the trauma experienced after Amy's birth when it was clear that Amy had Down syndrome. She recalled weeping in the hospital, and a well-intentioned nurse advised her that a mother was like a balloon that could go up or down; if down, she could pull the whole family down. With courage and love, this mother had decided to suppress her grief, to be that balloon soaring up. Now, some 24 years later, I was encouraging her to express grief in order to help her daughter.

Just before ending this initial meeting, Amy's mother remembered one further loss Amy had suffered. Some years before, at age 16, Amy's best friend, Lynn, died unexpectedly of heart disease. She had always been a weak child whose congenital heart condition demanded a quiet, sedentary lifestyle. Best friends for years, Amy and Lynn would play quietly and read together. Amy had attended Lynn's memorial service and had not appeared sad. It seemed to her family that she had accepted Lynn's death and that Lynn was in heaven. The accumulation of such losses must have had a staggering impact: a favorite peer dead, two siblings and a niece moved away from home. How could such a young woman handle the severe grief which she must have felt? Did the persistence of her silence signal a grief that had become arrested because this succession of losses was too great for her to bear?

~

Sessions with Amy ensued the week following my meeting with her mother. I wanted to plunge right in, building up a sense of identity and personal history and identifying feeling states with her. At my request, Amy came in with a photo album of family pictures to each of these initial sessions. Amy sat aloof and unresponsive while I looked at pictures and described what I saw. There were wonderful snapshots of Amy at home, at the beach, at parties. Pointing to each picture, I spoke about them to Amy. "There you are, Amy!" I did my best to describe the situation in each photo: who she was with, what was happening, whatever I guessed she might have been feeling. "You were playing on the beach, Amy. It looks like you were with your sister. You were smiling. You looked happy!" After seeing a number of pictures I added, "I'm wondering if you miss her. She got married and moved to her own home."

At the end of each session, Amy's mother joined us. She was invaluable in explaining more about the photos. We could talk in more depth about her memories of Amy. If I directed us toward feelings of loss, Amy's mother could talk about those feelings she had and that Amy might have had too. As conjoint sessions continued, Amy's mother remembered to bring up still more losses. Amy's grandparents had died in the past few years, and Amy's mother recalled how much Amy had enjoyed letters from them and that she would write back. While her mother talked about loss, Amy often raised her hands behind her head and waved her fingers. I commented to Amy that maybe she was telling us with her hands that she was upset, that she missed these people very deeply. Amy's mother shared her own observation that Amy waves her hands a great deal in church. I verbalized a hunch to Amy that she may feel sad in church, remembering funerals and remembering weddings that led to her brothers and sisters moving to their own homes. We talked too about friends who had moved away to out-of-state residential schools. I wondered out loud if Amy missed her friends and also if she worried that she would be sent away to a residential school. Amy's mother assured her daughter that she would always remain with or close to family.

In the room with this silent patient, I continued week after week to look through the scrapbooks. In addition to the photos I saw, I talked about people like Lynn and her grandparents whom I did not see pictures of, but suspected Amy missed very much. I talked about good times and about painful feelings when saying goodbye. Knowing that she seemed to hallucinate about God and that her family was devout, I voiced that she may have even felt angry at God for allowing these deaths. And she may have also felt angry at her sisters and brothers for leaving, especially with her brother for taking her niece, Carolyn, with him.

It was unsettling to talk at such length to a patient who appeared so detached while I spoke. While she generally did not look at me, I wondered if it was my imagination that she seemed to make a bit more eye contact with me before her eyes darted away. Her mother noticed a change at home. Amy had begun to gesture with a raised hand to indicate to her mother not to rush her when she did chores. Pleased to see her daughter asserting herself, Amy's mother backed off and told Amy she could have more time. As a result, Amy's mother soon noticed Amy doing more chores and doing them more willingly. Amy was not yet speaking, but she was beginning to communicate. I hoped we were on the right track.

The sudden loss of her friend Lynn was the focus to which I returned countless times. I retold stories I had been told of things they had done together and verbalized again and again how shocked she must have been when Lynn died. It was now almost time for Amy to leave for her summer vacation. There would be a 2-week break from therapy. Because of her potential to feel less connected to me when she returned, I wanted some indication about Amy's ability to relate to what I was saying about people who had been important to her. Was she hearing me, or was she absorbed in psychotic thinking as her aloofness might suggest? I asked Amy to tell me or write me a message about Lynn. I put a paper and pen on the desk. She reached slowly for the pen and took it hesitantly from my hand. She slowly bent over the paper, hesitated, and then printed a simple but clear message in her own phonetic way: "LYN DED." She then went on to write more but in words that I could not understand. This was her private language. But in these first two words, "LYN DED," she let me know that indeed she could relate to the grief that I had expressed to her. With her immediate shift from that thought about the death of her friend into private language, I could see her regression when overwhelmed with painful or confused feelings. Private language appeared for Amy to be a defense against sadness and fear rather than true psychotic thinking.

"LYN DED" was the first of what would be weekly letters that she spent each of her sessions writing in the months and years to follow. Each week Amy sat down and took out paper to write as soon as she came in. As she wrote, she occasionally said a word out loud, especially if I was at a loss to read her phonetic writing correctly. With the exception of this first letter, where I asked her to write or tell me about Lynn, Amy always initiated whom she wrote to and what she wrote about.

When Amy's mother came in, Amy read her letter about Lynn to her mother. Amy's mother and I talked more about Amy and Lynn's friendship, the heart condition, and the death. The following week, Amy wrote Lynn's name and a date, "JUNE 5." Amy could not explain the importance of this date. Her mother thought it might be the date when Lynn had died; I later learned this was not so but that date was connected in Amy's mind with Lynn. As we approached the anniversary of the June date the following year, it came up again in therapy. Amy's mother and I talked more about Lynn, how restricted the girls had been in activity because of Lynn's heart, and, again, the untimeliness and shock of her death. Amy was now hearing her grief validated.

Shortly thereafter, Amy's mother told me that Amy was changing more at home. She had resumed her prior practice of saying grace out loud at mealtime. And a couple of weeks later, Amy picked up an anniversary card that arrived for her parents and read it out loud to everyone just as she had done when she was younger.

~

Summer arrived, and it was time for Amy to leave for camp, followed by 2 weeks of family reunion and the celebration of Amy's birthday at the beach. Until recently, these summers had been happy times for Amy. Before she left, I wrote out a message for her and read it to her as I wrote. I wrote that I was glad she could have a vacation with her family and celebrate her birthday with them. In my letter I told her that I would miss her very much, but I knew she would be having a special time on vacation. To my surprise, Amy picked up my letter and read it out loud. I had never heard more than a word or two out loud while she was writing her weekly letters. Now I could hear her speaking for the first time as she read quickly and easily, speaking in a quiet monotone. She wanted to take my letter with her.

When Amy returned from vacation, her first letter, not surprisingly, was written totally in private language, which she would not explain. Even her handwriting deteriorated to a scrawl. But while she was undoubtedly reacting to the brief separation, her mother reported significant improvement over the vacation period. Amy had been much more like her old self, participating playfully in the pool instead of sitting on the edge. She kept up with the family when they took walks instead of holding back to walk alone. Alone with me for a minute while we moved from the clinic waiting room to my office, Amy's mother told me of a dream she had the night before. She dreamed that Amy had spoken to her. Clearly, Amy's withdrawal had been intensely painful for her family, and her mother was fully engaged in the process of helping Amy resume meaningful relationships. It was not long before Amy began a weekly ritual of reading the letters she wrote in therapy out loud to her mother as soon as her mother came in to join us.

A pattern emerged in her retreats into her incomprehensible, private language. It usually occurred immediately following breaks from therapy, when she was upset about being rushed in the morning before arriving at my office, if something unsettling had occurred, or in sessions immediately following ones where painful material came up in her letter. It seemed to occur when she felt lost, abandoned, angry, or frustrated.

Soon after her return from this first vacation, her messages became clearer and longer. She wrote two letters involving characters from the Wizard of Oz, one addressed to Aunt Em and one to Dorothy. She wrote that Dorothy was sitting on her bed feeling scared. Amy stopped writing. She could not respond to my questions: "What did Dorothy do?" "What was happening?" "What happened next?" Amy remained silent. Her expression looked worried. She bounced in her seat. She waved her fingers behind her head. I told Amy that, from her bouncing and her fingers, I thought she was upset. She still could not write further. Sensing that Amy's own scared feelings about separation and loss may have generated her focus on Dorothy, I proceeded on a hunch, going with the pilot line of the story at this critical point. I spoke to Amy about the story of Dorothy swept up into the sky, away from the people she loved the most, her aunt and uncle. I wondered if Amy might feel a lot like Dorothy, losing people like her friend Lynn who died, her grandparents who died, and her sisters, brothers, and niece who moved. Amy still did not write, but continued to bounce. Her eyes looked frightened. Finally, I asked Amy if we could take care of Dorothy. At this point Amy wrote: "I HER FREND." Amy's ability to empathize with Dorothy was startling in light of her apparent detachment.

This was not the last time that Amy addressed or wrote about fictional characters. When asked if they were real or from stories, she could always write with certainty or acknowledge with a nod of the head that they were stories. Feeling fairly sure that her thinking was not psychotic, I saw that we could use these fictional characters in therapy to allow Amy an easier way to express issues and feelings that were central to her own life. I felt safe joining her in the fiction, seeing that this brought her closer to reality rather than escaping from it.

"AMY SHE DED" was the frightening statement in her next letter following the Wizard of Oz letters. Again she could go no further, and again I tried to stay with her and expressed a hunch. I wondered if Amy wanted to be dead in order to be in heaven with the people she missed. Amy began bouncing in her chair but could not write. When her mother came in, Amy read her letter out loud to her mother. "Amy she ded" brought back memories to her mother. When Lynn and her grandparents died, Amy had said, "Amy gone to Heaven." Amy's mother talked more with us about her memories of the deaths and the funerals. She remembered Amy putting her hand in her grandmother's at the viewing and how she had run out of the room crying.

Amy retreated into science fiction in the letters immediately following these painful letters about death. She waved her fingers behind her head, bounced in her chair, tapped her pen. I reminded her that we had been writing and talking about some very important but difficult events: her friend's death, her grandparents' death, and how it may have felt to lose these people. Amy began waving her fingers behind her head more than I had seen her do for a long time. I pointed this out and wondered if she was thinking of angels in heaven when she flapped her fingers. "Um hmm" she agreed. Sometimes Amy agrees to things that I later find out are not factually incorrect, but since she can say a very definite "NO!" to some things, I cannot help but wonder if the "yes" might be at least an indication that some part of what she is agreeing to strikes her as true. Again I was not certain if her thinking was psychotic regarding "Amy she ded." I asked her if she was with God in heaven or here with Mom and Dad. She answered quickly that she was with her parents.

~

It was only a couple of weeks before Amy returned to the topic of Lynn and her other school friends. Fragmented ideas emerged about kids fighting at school. This was in a religious context. "Bad thing,"

Amy wrote, and "Jesus cries." There was no explanation for why Jesus would cry. I asked Amy if she was worried that she had done some bad thing herself. She began writing about fights at school. Lynn, she wrote, had pushed a boy in the street: "bad push . . . Amy up wall." She wrote names of kids who had been involved. I repeated that Lynn had pushed and gave permission to the idea that Amy might have felt angry and even pushed back. Even if a friend is ill, it is hard for kids to always remember to be gentle and careful. Amy came back to this topic some months later when she wrote that she and Lynn ran fast. Perhaps Amy blamed herself for causing Lynn's death by running fast with her, a forbidden activity due to Lynn's heart condition. Possibly her silence was her way of keeping her part in Lynn's death a secret. Amy seemed more connected to me once she began writing about these fights in school that had occurred many years ago. She waved her hands less and even addressed one of her letters to me.

She wrote that she was thinking about herself talking. Now she shifted to writing for the first time of a current concern, different from the early letters she wrote of events in the distant past. "Feel sad . . . miss somebody. . . ." She stopped writing for quite some time, leaned forward toward me, squinted, and stared intently at me but wrote no more. "You want me to understand, don't you, Amy?" With encouragement and questions she finally told me it was her father she was missing but could not tell me why. When her mother joined us, she filled in what Amy could not explain: that Amy's father had left the night before for a trip out of town. We talked together about missing him. Amy continued to show more progresss at home. In recent years, Amy had been silent when she returned home each day from her sheltered workshop and her mother asked about her day. To her mother's surprise and pleasure, Amy now began answering, albeit briefly.

Therapy became a place where Amy could address important issues and participate in making decisions. The first time this happened, Amy's mother raised her own uncertainty about where to sign Amy up for sleep-away summer camp. Unsure where Amy felt happiest, her mother reviewed the options. Amy gave strong preferences with body language: angry, scared expressions, and a firm "No!" or a nod of consent as we spent weeks going over the choices. When this topic came up the following spring, it was again time for Amy to choose. She wrote about camp, then shifted to writing about Jack the Ripper. I asked her if Jack the Ripper was her way of telling us that she was scared of something happening to her at camp. She nodded in agreement that she was scared, wrote that something happened in the cabin, but could write no more. I tried to elicit more information about who was in the cabin with her or what had happened but she was unable to respond then or later when I attempted to come back to the scary episode in the cabin. Rather than pressing her for details she seemed unable to share, I concluded that whatever the episode, it was too painful for her to deal with it. Despite the fact that I was working partly in the dark, I moved on to talk with her about ways she could be assertive at camp next summer if anything happened that frightened her. I role-played how she could say "no" or physically move away from anyone who might make her feel uncomfortable. I asked if she would like me to write a letter to her camp director that she could keep in her suitcase in case she got scared. She nodded and seemed glad to have it. I read the letter out loud to Amy as I wrote it, explaining to the director that if Amy brought this letter to her it meant she was upset or scared and in need of help. The following year when she wrote about packing for camp, she seemed quite upset, eyes frightened and waving her hands behind her head, until I asked if she wanted another letter for the new director. She wanted it, and I gave her one. Although we never did find out what had happened in the cabin that had frightened her, we were able to identify the scary feeling and help her cope with it. These annual camp decisions were an important time in therapy during which she had the experience of making large decisions after her opinions were carefully solicited and weighed.

When Amy resumed speaking out loud in the first year of therapy, her short statements, often one isolated word, were always said in anger. In one of the first, she let her family know that she did not want to miss a stopover at a certain fast food restaurant when they were on the highway. These angry verbalizations continued as her exclusive way of communicating for over a year. With great understanding, her family accepted and welcomed her words, however angry, learning that her anger was a necessary part of her emerging from a world where she had felt alone and frightened.

Amy continued to use her weekly letters to address issues of concern, especially about situations where she had felt scared. She increasingly wrote of episodes that had happened in the week prior to seeing me. Now she could write about something fresh on her mind. One week she wrote about her mother working in the kitchen, and a pot burning on the stovetop. She had been scared and wrote to her mother to be careful. Another week she wrote in a very indirect way about a "lieutenant." When I asked what "lieutenant" Amy could be thinking of, her mother remembered that Amy had been separated from her group on a recent field trip out of state to an amusement park and had needed the help of a security guard. Even her mother had not realized how scared Amy had been until we went over this letter. I turned to Amy and asked if her mother and I were on the right track. I asked

Amy if she used the word "lieutenant" to tell us that she needed protection from someone like a guard or policeman. She gave a quick, sharp nod of agreement. Her mother and I then went on to talk about how scary it must have been to get lost in a huge amusement park and the need to find someone to help. Amy's mother and I both were able to give Amy feedback that she had handled a difficult situation very well. From this session on, I knew that if Amy used the word "lieutenant," I should ask if something scary had happened and she needed protection; the word "lieutenant" became her shortcut way of telling me she needed protection on a number of different occasions.

~

At the time of this writing, Amy is 27 years old and we are completing 3 years of psychotherapy. It is significant that, in psychological testing done this spring, she drew a picture of herself and her mother in the projective part of the testing. Two circles next to each other were identified as herself and her mother, with a large rectangle underneath meant to be a table. It is telling that this patient, emerging from years of silence, described the picture with one word: "discussion."

Amy's mother has just undergone major back surgery. This could have been a frightening crisis for Amy, and we used therapy to prepare her and to learn what she felt about it. She wrote "scared." When asked if she was scared about what would be happening to her mother or happening to herself, she wrote "Amy." She wrote that she was scared of being alone. Amy's mother and I talked about how different it would be with Mother in the hospital and then with Mother home but resting in bed most of the time. Her mother reassured Amy that other family members would be there for her. Amy agreed that her mother could let them know that she was scared and needed their help and understanding. Amy handled the surgery and her mother's convalescence surprisingly well. The week after surgery, she wrote a letter while her mother was still in the hospital: ". . . thinking about Mom in hospital . . . body . . . big knife . . . miss her a lot. . . ."

In this last year, Amy has begun speaking to her family without the constant angry undertone that had punctuated the few words she said in the first 2 years of therapy. Now she shows us a wider range of feelings in her speech. "I'd like an egg," Amy said recently to her mother and sister to their delight. This simple sentence revealed great progress: "I"—a pronoun reclaiming a regained sense of self; "I'd like"—telling us that she is beginning to identify a feeling state on her own, a need; "I'd like an egg"—an ability to formulate a complete and clear statement allowing her to reconnect with her family and have her needs met. Amy is coming out of "cold storage."

Soon after this exchange, she wrote a letter addressed to her mother, whom she now calls "Mother" again, retreating to "Pam" only when she feels very alone.

> Dear mother
> I like go walk
> dosit sonwon
> eveinanwd
> neighborhood
> watto to eat
> lucher

She wrote this, as always, in her own phonetic way, asking for help with spelling the hardest word, "neighborhood." As she wrote, she read it slowly out loud: "Dear Mother, I like go for a walk . . . soon . . . evening . . . around the neighborhood . . . want to eat . . . lunch." Amy and her mother can now resume two favorite activities together.

REFERENCES

Rako, S., & Mazer, H. (1980). *Semrad: The heart of a therapist.* Northvale, NJ: Jason Aronson, Inc.

Tustin, F. (1986). *Autistic barriers in neurotic patients.* New Haven, CT: Yale University Press.

11

Glimpses of Lives

Stories of Brief Treatment

Mary Ann Blotzer

Sometimes our work with patients is brief, perhaps because the patient only needs some short-term work around a focal issue that is soon resolved. In these cases, therapy ends with a sense of completeness. At other times external factors impinge on the treatment: A patient loses the insurance that pays for treatment, or transportation problems become so overwhelming that the patient literally cannot get to treatment. These situations leave us feeling disappointed or frustrated, regretting unfulfilled possibilities, saying to ourselves, "if only" or "what if."

Nevertheless, brief treatment, whether brief because the work is soon completed or because external factors prevented completion, is a fact of life. Lessons can be learned in both sets of circumstances. What follows here are brief glimpses into lives. Some feel complete. Others haunt me still today.

~

Ralph: A Story of Loss and Reclamation Occasionally our patients show us precisely what they need. Such was the case with Ralph, a man in his 50s who had severe mental retardation. Until 6 months prior to seeing me, he had lived a cozy, if constricted, life with his elderly mother. Ralph's father had died many years before; a younger sister of Ralph's, Sheila, lived an hour's drive away with her husband and their three teenagers.

From Sheila's description, I pictured Ralph and his mother living as an old married couple. They seldom went anywhere and spent their time companionably puttering around the house together. Despite being in her 70s, Ralph's mother still cooked the evening meal. Together she and Ralph would clean up afterward and settle in for an evening of television watching. Although Sheila had often urged her mother to have Ralph attend some type of day or work program, both Ralph and the mother refused. They enjoyed their cloistered existence. But that cloistered existence came to an abrupt end when Ralph's mother died in her sleep one evening. As best we can piece together, Ralph became concerned when his mother was not at breakfast the next morning and went to her room, where he tried in vain to wake her. Alarmed, he ran to a neighbor, who returned to the house and took charge of the situation. Within the day, Ralph left his lifelong home and moved in with his sister, her husband, and their children. He was never to return again to the family home.

Emergencies, by their very nature, leave us with no time to plan. And under stress, we have less emotional energy available to weigh our needs and options. Sheila was a kind woman who cared deeply about her brother, but given her own grief and the demands of her children she had neither the time nor the emotional energy to consider how to ease the transition for Ralph. A combination of factors led to her decision to exclude Ralph from his mother's funeral and to never sit down with Ralph to discuss his mother's death. Because Ralph lacked the expressive language abilities to formulate his concerns, Sheila only fleetingly considered that he might be full of unexpressed questions and feelings. It was also emotionally easier for her to take this approach. Her own grief was painful enough to her. She feared being overwhelmed by both her own and her brother's grief; she also feared that eliciting his feelings would make matters worse. What if he became terribly distraught and she could not calm him down?

These issues are not uncommon. Persons with intellectual disabilities or expressive language problems may lack the ability to articulate their thoughts clearly. It is not as though they walk into our offices and say, "I'm depressed since my mother died, and I've lots of worries for the future." Ralph's difficulty communicating colluded with his sister's reluctance to discuss painful, emotionally charged material to formulate the family belief that Ralph had no feelings about the loss of his mother and the abrupt transitions he was forced to make. Even when caregivers sense that the person is troubled, they may feel deeply inadequate about their ability to help the person. The painful irony is that closing the door on emotionally laden material in the hopes of protection usually has the opposite effect. It leaves the person alone with his fears and fantasies and with no opportunity for feedback. This isolation can be a recipe for deterioration into psychotic symptoms.

Ralph and his family were referred to me approximately 6 months after his mother's death. Ralph had been steadily deteriorating. He was becoming increasingly withdrawn, barely responding to others, and spending most of his time in a rocking chair in a corner of the family room, staring out the window, seemingly oblivious to those around him. Most alarmingly, he was barely eating and was steadily losing weight. Grasping at straws, Sheila decided to follow the advice of her family doctor and pursue therapy for Ralph, despite being dubious that someone with severe mental retardation and minimal speech could engage in therapy. Numerous practical realities impinged on the case, a common situation in the lives of persons with disabilities and their families. Because of inadequate health insurance to cover therapy and an already overcommitted family that did not have time in its schedule to drive Ralph to therapy on a weekly basis, we agreed that I would see Ralph for a two- to four-session extended evaluation to develop an assessment and recommendations. I could hear the relief in Sheila's voice when I suggested this brief approach. She was already overwhelmed, and the thought of a long stretch of therapy with its attendant demands on her was more than she could realistically handle.

I remember being startled when I met Ralph. He seemed spectral—pale, gaunt, his clothes hanging on his frame—and he followed me wordlessly and impassively into my office. So incorporeal did he seem that I remember having the fantasy that my hand would pass through his as we shook hands. Literally and metaphorically, Ralph seemed to be fading from existence, gradually disappearing into nothingness. We spent a few minutes silently tuning ourselves to one another. I matched my breathing to his and was careful not to look too directly at him or to overwhelm him in any way. I sensed that I could easily overwhelm him if I were too alive. After a little while, he seemed both more alert and more relaxed. While Ralph sat silently, I pondered aloud about what he might be going through, giving voice to that which he felt but could not express. He looked alertly at me a few times as I did this. I held his gaze only briefly before looking away again. Then he picked up the pillow from his chair, held it in front of his face, and slowly peered out at me from one side of the pillow. Taking his lead, I followed along in this version of peek-a-boo. I said, "Peek-a-boo, I see you." Something in Ralph resonated to this, so I repeated again, with more animation, "I see you," as Ralph alternately hid behind and peered out from the pillow that he was holding in front of his face. And then I quietly said, "Perhaps with your mother dead, you feel as though no one sees you anymore, as though you're becoming dead." Wordlessly, Ralph's eyes filled with tears.

The infant is born psychologically, as a separate person, through seeing himself reflected in his mother's responses to him. Colloquially, we have many phrases for acknowledging this—"the apple of his mother's eye," and our reference to the time even before birth, "when you were just a gleam in your mother's eye." The philosophical conundrum, "Does a tree falling in the forest make any sound if no one is there to hear it?" reflects this concern as well. Do we exist if no one is there to acknowledge our existence? To be deeply and accurately known by another human being is perhaps our most compelling psychological need. In Ralph's case, feeling unknown was keeping him from eating enough to stay alive. Ralph had been the apple of his mother's eye, but the apple tree had died, and Ralph was going to die too unless he could again see himself in the reflected glory of another's eyes.

I saw Ralph only a few times, and I chatted briefly with Sheila on each of these occasions. Twice the three of us met together to talk about Ralph's fears and worries. I included Sheila in this because I wanted to model a way to talk with Ralph about these issues, and I sensed that Sheila would feel more secure about future talks with Ralph if we first tried this together in the safety of my office. Ralph had an associational and tangential way of responding in conversation that made it difficult for the uninitiated to follow his meaning. Most individuals follow a conversation in a more linear fashion, building upon the topic. Ralph, largely due to his limits, responded in an associational fashion, finding some element of the conversation that he could connect with and taking it from there. Although "there" seldom seemed to follow the theme, it did reveal important clues about Ralph's concerns. Sheila, being perceptive, quickly recognized in our work together that what Ralph said was not bizarre and meaningless but rather reflected his best efforts to connect with us. She learned that by following Ralph's lead and by thinking in a more associational and metaphorical fashion she could meaningfully talk with Ralph about his feelings.

Ralph steadily returned to the land of the living as his concerns were given voice in therapy and addressed in daily life with his family. He began to enjoy food and other pleasures again. When he says, "Miss mom," Sheila responds with an empathetic acknowledgment. In some ways, he has replicated the cozy yet constricted life that he led with his mother before her death. He has resisted Sheila's encouragement to participate in a day or work program. He prefers instead to help Sheila around the house and to occasionally help neighbors with their yard work. This narrow life satisfies him. He prefers the world of family and neighborhood to the bustle of work and has demonstrated the contributions that he can make in these realms.

Recently, Sheila phoned me to say that an elderly neighbor of theirs, Sam, had lost his wife. Upon being told of this, Ralph said, "Sam's sad. I'm sad." And having seen Sheila on numerous occasions take casseroles to recently bereaved families, Ralph opened their refrigerator and pulled out a six pack of blueberry yogurt (his favorite) and announced to Sheila that he was taking this to Sam.

~

Frances: A Case of Suspended Animation The *Diagnostic and Statistical Manual of Mental Disorders* (fourth edition) *(*DSM-IV*)* (American Psychiatric Association, 1994) divides the disorders into type. The manual includes a section on mood disorders, on personality disorders, and on disorders usually first diagnosed in infancy, childhood, and adolescence. It even includes a section, "Mental Disorders Due to a General Medical Condition." I have often thought that there ought to be a section of DSM-IV devoted to disorders caused by failures of the social contract. Although mental health is always affected by the adequacy of social supports, the relationship is especially strong where persons with disabilities are concerned. Adequate attendant care, accessible housing and transportation, and laws such as the Americans with Disabilities Act (PL 101-336) that guarantee fair employment practices enable persons with disabilities to live in the community, hold down a job and receive the financial and personal benefits that accrue from employment, and enjoy social relationships, including sexual relationships. Without these supports, vibrant, capable adults are forced to live constricted lives in nursing homes. Almost everything— employment, community living, and strong social relationships— hinges on adequate services and legal protections.

This dependency is perhaps even greater for persons with mental retardation as they seek to make the transition to adult roles. Although federal law guarantees appropriate educational services through age 21, there are no service entitlements after this age. The collision between developmental imperatives and inadequate social supports could not be more striking. Just when young adults are seeking greater independence from their families, they are forced into a position of even greater dependency. Their families, already worn down by years of caregiving, see only a bleak future ahead. While their peers who have children without disabilities are enjoying increasing freedom and pride at seeing their adult children launched into the world, parents of young adults with disabilities face added caregiving demands. Many mothers are forced to abandon their careers because their adult children no longer have a place to go during the day. They are deprived of one of the great satisfactions of parenthood: seeing their children settled and secure. Instead, as one mother said to me, "I feel like I'm not allowed to die."

The combined stresses upon parents and their adult children often result in the development of mental disorders. Unfortunately, it is not uncommon to see young adults who had functioned well throughout their school years suddenly appear in mental health clinics with serious disorders: major depression, depression with psychotic features, elective mutism, and anorexia nervosa, to name a few. They develop these disorders because they are not given the services they need to make the successful transition into adult roles. The lack of appropriate adult services leaves them stranded in a state of suspended animation, no longer children but unable to achieve adult roles and autonomy without help. Such was Frances's story.

Frances was nearly mute when she appeared in my office. Her parents brought her to treatment only when a former teacher ran into Frances and was alarmed at the depth of her withdrawal and urged the parents to seek mental health treatment. Frances stayed in her room all day, never initiated conversation, and when queried would respond only in barely audible monosyllables. Her parents reported that she had an imaginary friend she would talk to.

I found it painful to sit with Frances. Her downcast eyes, lethargic movements, and minimal responsiveness radiated depression more powerfully than other depressed patients whom I had seen. At age 25 she seemed to have given up completely and retreated to a semi-vegetative existence. Equally painful to watch were Frances's parents. They had helplessly watched Frances's decline without alarm. Lacking confidence that things could be different, they waited nearly a year before bringing Frances to treatment and did so only because of her former teacher's shock at the change in her.

That made two of us who felt alarmed. Alvarez (1992) has written about the alarm that therapists sometimes feel when treating seriously regressed patients. She describes the reclamatory functions of the therapist as he or she tries to pull the patient back into a sense of connectedness. In the treatment room with Frances and her parents, I felt a sense of urgency to try to activate both Frances and her parents. What had happened to their alarm, and why was I feeling all of it?

The details of Frances's deterioration were emblematic of all the inadequacies of our public policy toward adults with mental retardation and the families that care for them. During the latter years of her schooling, Frances was placed in a job. Someone from her school, a job coach, checked on her regularly and met with her supervisor to troubleshoot. In this way, problems were caught early and corrected. Both Frances and her supervisor felt supported. The job continued after Frances's graduation along with the services of the job coach. Frances seemed happy. She had a reason to get out of bed in the morning, a structure to her life, and a job that gave her social outlets and some sense of satisfaction.

Unfortunately, according to government policy, funding for the job coach ended one year after Frances's graduation. Frances's parents tried to fill in. They met periodically with Frances's supervisor, who reported that Frances was not working as diligently as she should now that the job coach was gone. Frances's parents encouraged her and exhorted her to do better, but this was not enough. Frances needed more support on the job. Although the supervisor said that Frances needed to work harder, he never threatened adverse action. Frances and her parents were left thinking that the job was secure. Abruptly, Frances was fired. She came home one day with a note telling her parents not to send her back.

Mr. and Mrs. P tried in vain to find another job for their daughter. Their dealings with the vocational rehabilitation agency were demoralizing. Not wanting to give them false hope, the vocational rehabilitation counselor gave them no hope. Without the structure of a job and without hope, Frances began a steady deterioration, culminating in her appearance in my office, meeting all the diagnostic criteria for depression with psychotic features. But I found myself wanting to add another axis on the diagnostic form, "Disorder caused by failure of social policy."

Because of scheduling limitations, I was unable to see Frances and referred her to a colleague who also specialized in this type of work and who I knew would also assist Mr. and Mrs. P at advocating for their daughter with the vocational rehabilitation agency. But Frances's story and the hopelessness that her parents felt haunts me still today, fueling my activism. In figurative terms, they projected all of their alarm into me, and I remain committed to arousing the same alarm in policy makers.

~

Diane: Neither "Super-Crip" nor Poster Child Persons with disabilities have much to be angry about: anger at their disability, anger at the barriers and failures of accommodation that they encounter, and sometimes even anger at themselves for feeling angry. The demands of managing this anger extract an enormous toll. It is never simple, as the individual's beliefs and conflicts about aggression, about the legitimacy of his anger, about what our culture expects from persons with disabilities, and about a host of other issues combine into a murky morass that complicates both the internal perception and outward expression of anger. Olkin (1993), writing about the pressures that are placed upon persons with disabilities to regulate their affect in ways acceptable to others, has coined the term *decontextualized rage*:

> I strongly believe that there are two groups in America whose anger is never tolerated, accepted, or perhaps understood: young black males and people with disabilities. Both share the problem of a) decontextualized rage, i.e., rage seen as a response to a single event, rather than to a greater social context; b) a view of rage as a violation of the desired (not actual) norm set for their group; and c) a definition of rage for their social group as indicative of individual pathology, lack of adjustment, and failure to be appropriately socialized. (p. 14)

The disability experience is still so poorly understood, and persons with disabilities the objects of so much distortion, fantasy, and projection, that their reactions are typically viewed under the lens of how the majority culture needs them to respond. Failure to meet these expectations is usually greeted with disapprobation. Legitimate anger at barriers and failures of accommodation, as well as anger at condescending treatment, is viewed as pathology. When persons with disabilities object to demeaning portrayals on telethons or other fund-raising events that portray them as objects of pity or charity, they are viewed as ungrateful and mean spirited. Don't they appreciate the good intentions behind the fund-raiser? Can't they politely behave like good little poster children?

But the realm of therapy is the intersection between subjective reality and the external world. Perhaps there is no better setting than the therapeutic relationship for persons with disabilities to explore the intersection between unjust, condescending, bigoted treatment and their own mix of feelings, conflicts, fantasies, and wishes about this treatment. Such was the work of Diane's therapy.

As fate would have it, Diane's first appointment with me occurred after a major snowfall. Diane, who has cerebral palsy, uses a motorized wheelchair. In banking up the snow, the plows had managed to cover most of the ramps in the area surrounding my office. Finding a passable route to my building was a frustrating, time-consuming ordeal, and Diane only made it into the building with assistance from two passersby who literally lifted her chair over a snow-packed curb. Although she appreciated their assistance, this independent woman felt demeaned at having been forced into such a position. Patients are especially vulnerable when they first begin therapy. The awareness that perhaps they need assistance intensifies all their vulnerabilities surrounding such loaded issues as dependency, autonomy, and their own adequacy and worth. Diane's already heightened vulnerability was further bruised at literally having to ask for help to even enter my office.

And so it was that she arrived late for her first appointment with me, with all these issues brimming up inside her. A meticulously organized woman who prided herself on her punctuality, she was made late because the route was impassable. She was physically exhausted and emotionally frustrated by the numerous unsuccessful attempts she had made to get into the building under her own power. But like most individuals, she wanted to put her best foot forward in her first meeting with me. Caught between exhaustion, frustration, and her desire to make a good impression, she felt doubly frustrated at being forced into this untenable position by unthinking snowplow operators who consider ramps convenient places to pile snow. She was also angry at me. I had been recommended as someone with expertise in disabilities, yet I had failed to notify her that the route from the parking lot to my building was impassable by wheelchair. At the same time, she did not feel that she could safely vent this anger in her first meeting with me. Would I, a member of the mental health profession, pathologize her if her anger was too raw and unfiltered? If she expressed it in a controlled, modulated fashion, would I still think that any anger signified her lack of "adjustment?" Was it even "fair" of her to think that I should have notified her, or was she trying to be a "super crip" by insisting on traveling in such bad weather? (The words in quotation marks are the words that Diane used when we later discussed her conflicts on that day.)

The effort of sitting on this mix of feelings made for a stilted few minutes as we settled in with one another, both wondering what to expect. She was angry, tearful, and struggling to maintain her composure as we discussed her predicament trying to enter the building. "Those f-ing snowplow operators, someone ought to strand them in a parking lot for hours! Don't they know what they're doing to us?" Sensing that she was also angry at me and wondering whether I (like the snowplow driver) knew what I was doing "to her," I wondered aloud if she was also angry at me for not alerting her to the impassable ramps. She immediately responded to this, and we productively discussed both her expectations of others and her conflicts about these expectations. Were her expectations "fair?" Did they overwhelm others? How could she best communicate them? Should she even have to communicate them? How would others receive her? Over the next several weeks we dove wholeheartedly into these issues, into the anger that inevitably was triggered when her expectations were violated and the ways in which she managed this anger.

In an early session, she related a story that was classic in the bigotry that it reflected and in the dilemmas that it presented her with. Having recently moved to the Washington, D.C., area and eager to meet people, she enrolled in an adult education class. She arrived early and had begun chatting with the other students. She was feeling comfortable and included. Suddenly, the instructor strode purposefully into the room, took one look at Diane in her wheelchair, and perkily announced, "Oh, I see we have a very special student!" It was an inanely gratuitous comment motivated by discomfort, and it singled Diane out. She could no longer be just a member of the class. Fueling Diane's outrage and frustration was her sense that she had to respond with a gracious smile lest she be viewed as "just a nasty, maladjusted crip." Diane went on, "What I really wanted to say was, 'Oh, I see we have a very condescending instructor.'" We enjoyed a rich laugh at the prospect of responding with this or with the current euphemism, "an attitudinally challenged instructor." But when our laughter abated we were left with Diane's rage, its accretions and distortions, and her conflicts about that rage.

Diane told me that given her penchant for expressing herself with four-letter words, a friend had dubbed her "Queen of the 'F' word." She knew that the intensity of her anger often seemed disproportionate to the precipitant and that her intense expressions of anger sometimes drove people away from her. Her anger had multiple determinants reaching far back into her history.

Born in the early 1960s, she was the middle of three children in a middle-class Jewish family. Her father owned a hardware store in a Southern city where few other Jewish families lived. Bright and competitive, she resented the roles assigned her by disability and gender. Although significantly brighter than her older brother, her parents encouraged her brother's academic aspirations, but not hers. Diane described her younger sister as a "piece of fluff" who was expected to look pretty and marry someone who would support her. Diane described her family as "not knowing what to do with me." She was an intelligent girl in a family that only nurtured intelligence in boys, and she was a physically imperfect girl in a family that valued physical perfection in its girls. But above all, this family only two generations removed from the shetl valued fitting in with its suburban neighbors and worked frantically to be a model of assimilation. Diane's father was tirelessly affable even when enduring unreasonable demands from customers. As a child, Diane spent much of her free time at her father's store. At times she thought he demeaned himself with his relentless affability and would ask him about this. He would reply that as a shopkeeper and minority he needed to "make nice" and encouraged her to do the same.

Diane grew up in a family that quickly "shushed" her if she expressed any anger or discontent or acted in ways counter to the prescribed code for Southern womanhood. Although she felt that her family was unreasonable in its expectations for conformity and rigid regulation of affect, she lacked confidence in the legitimacy of her feelings. As soon as she could, she moved away from her family. At the small women's college that she attended, her intellectual abilities were respected and her leadership skills were supported. After college, she moved to Maryland and took a job with a federal agency. It was there that she made her first connections with the disability rights movement and found others who validated her thinking. She was doing well.

Perhaps her doing well was what enabled her to initiate therapy. She had enough confidence in herself to address what had always been a nagging issue for her: the residue of her childhood conflicts about aggression and how this played out for her as an adult woman with a disability. It takes both discomfort and courage to begin therapy. Discomfort provides the necessary motivation, and courage is required to forthrightly examine oneself. Diane had both these factors in good measure. The intense, disproportionate way in which sometimes she expressed her anger left her feeling disappointed in herself and had also caused her problems at work.

Diane and I worked together for a little more than 6 months. That was all the time that she needed to examine what evoked her anger, her conflicts about its "legitimacy," and strategies for managing her anger that left her feeling that she had stood up for herself without being an aggressor. She needed very little from me as her therapist to facilitate this work. Mostly, she needed me to listen to her without "shushing" her when she would vent her rage and to acknowledge that her anger was understandable. This empathetic listening settled Diane sufficiently so that she could examine the intensity of her anger and alternatives for expressing it. Our time-limited work together illustrated the oscillation between the elements of psychoanalytically oriented and supportive psychotherapy, an oscillation that other chapters in this book have discussed. In psychoanalytic terms, I "contained" her anger so that she could better metabolize it. We would talk through why she felt it so intensely and then move to a practical discussion of ways to express her anger that left her feeling that she was "neither doormat nor aggressor." A woman of many strengths and good insight, Diane was able to resolve this issue in less than a year. Our work felt complete.

REFERENCES

Alvarez, A. (1992). *Live company: Psychoanalytic psychotherapy with autistic, borderline, deprived and abused children*. London: Routledge.

American Psychiatric Association. (1994). *Diagnostic and statistical manual of mental disorders* (4th ed.). Washington, DC: Author.

Americans with Disabilities Act of 1990, PL 101-336. (July 26, 1990). Title 42, U.S.C. 12101 et seq: *U.S. Statutes at Large, 104*, 327–378.

Olkin, R. (1993). Crips, gimps, and epileptics explain it all for you. *Readings: A Journal of Reviews and Commentary in Mental Health, 8*(4), 13–17.

12

Nancy Rainbow

A Case Study

Donald Cassidy

Nancy Rainbow was referred to me through a colleague who knew that I had a telecommunications device for the deaf (TDD) and that I had some experience working with Deaf cultural awareness and issues. My first meeting with her was by phone. I usually prefer meeting people in person. But a wise mentor once encouraged me to understand that therapy begins with the very first human contact, even if it is brief and appears to deal primarily with the logistics of where and when to meet in person.

My first impression of Nancy was the power of her words. She seemed bright, angry, humorous, anxious, and depressed. She communicated all of this without her voice via a TDD, because her hearing aids were broken and were not functional for phone use even when they did work. Despite the humor and power in her words, there was evidence of pain. She explained that, at her current age of 51, osteopetrosis had progressively robbed her of her hearing and some sight and caused her to be anemic. She had never learned to walk because her legs had not developed sufficiently to support her weight even with double canes or a walker. She had used a manual wheelchair for many years but now had a motorized one because, as she said, "sometimes I just like to get up a lot of speed and mow people down . . . ha ha, not really . . . but you know what I mean." In addition, she suffered from respiratory problems on a regular basis. Despite these disabilities, she and her husband had moved from Kansas to Washington, D.C., in order to be closer to advocacy and lobbying efforts for changes in federal policy and various kinds of legislation to help ensure the eventual passage of the Americans with Disabilities Act (ADA).

She stated that she sought supportive counseling for some of the difficult issues she faced on a daily basis, but I sensed that our work together would eventually also involve concentrated effort at helping her to deal with some of the accumulated anxiety and depression of a lifetime of discrimination and barriers. Although there is some controversy over whether hearing loss is a disability, I feel that the most important thing for me to do as a therapist is to help the individuals I am working with to clarify for themselves whether they experience their relative ability to hear as a "challenge," a "disability," or whatever words they wish to use. As a hearing person who works therapeutically with people who have hearing loss, I do not have a pre-set notion of which of these paradigms is more empowering for any given client who walks through the door of my office. I do believe that it is important to be aware of the tension between the symbolism of these two (and perhaps other) positions and to allow that to be therapeutic grist for the mill.

~

We agreed to meet for the first time at her home where she resided with her husband and two cats. I imagined that she wanted to assess my level of compassion, my awareness of disability rights issues, and my ability to communicate in American Sign Language (ASL). "Besides, I'm tired of always having to go to get help. This time I'd like for it to come to me. Do you make house calls, doc?" She went on to explain that she wanted me to see what her world was like before we discussed whether we were a good therapeutic team. She also wanted me to meet her husband.

In our first meeting, she told me that Nancy Rainbow was not her real name. She had changed it for several reasons. The main reason, she said, was that rainbows are God's way of transforming the gloom of a rainy day into something beautiful to behold through the use of the power of the light. Changing her first name to "Nancy" did not have any symbolic significance, as far as she knew; she just liked the name. Nancy was a deeply spiritual person, and it was clear that spirituality would not only be a theme in our work, but also a powerful force in the healing process. She also talked through some painful memories of growing up with multiple, progressively disabling physical conditions in a family of origin that was verbally abusive and not supportive of her needs. The choice of a new name was a proactive step to empower herself; it was also a way of leaving behind some painful memories.

The initial session went well. Her husband seemed interested in who I was and in my credentials. Another controversial issue in this work involved the use of ASL, signed English, and total communication. I explained that I try to tailor my communication style to the person I work with in order to facilitate trust and communication. Total communication (TC) using ASL and spoken English is a challenge because of the tremendous difference in syntax in the two languages and the necessity to think simultaneously in both. I explained that the only position I feel passionately about is that it is my job to find out which mode of communication is best for me to use for each individual client and then to let our linguistic differences either interfere as little as possible or to let them be material for therapy.

Although Nancy also spoke of some couples issues from her marriage, she was quite clear that she did not want to do couples work in this counseling. We discussed issues such as health insurance, fees, and the scope of the work. The insurance issue was easy because she had used her lifetime maximum benefits in all areas of coverage. She did not want me to do this work pro bono. She did have a modest income and wanted to pay me $10 per session.

I explained my background and training as a therapist, and Nancy seemed satisfied. My skills with ASL were less impressive. Typical of hearing people, my expressive skills far outshined my receptive skills. However, by using TC, Nancy and I were able to understand each other well enough. My credentials in Deaf cultural awareness, including coursework at Gallaudet College, life experience working as a counselor with people with hearing impairments, and other life experiences working with deaf and hearing-impaired people tipped the balance; we decided to work together. She suggested that my expressive skills would come in handy for doing some interpreting for her at workshops.

The initial phone/TDD session had apparently established a basis of hope. This first face-to-face session established a basis of communication and the beginnings of a level of trust. But it was the third session that seemed to be the one where we found each other as counselor and client. She was quite clear that she did not want me to be a therapist or a doctor. Since my theoretical orientation at that time was an eclectic blend of philosophy and skills that a graduate school mentor once described as being "eclectic–Jungian–Rogerian," I believed that I could be a competent counselor for Nancy.

~

During this third session she told me her "story." This was the history that I usually ask for in the first session with clients. However, we had done well to be patient and to spend the first two sessions discovering each other's levels of awareness and finding out whether we would work well together.

Nancy was the older of two children born to an angry, passive, alcoholic father who punished his family through a combination of verbally abusive outbursts and neglectful silent withdrawal. Her mother tried to hold the family together by sheer force of will, working as a bus driver to help support the family and trying to keep peace in the family. She was a strong, intelligent woman who was Nancy's role model for meeting life's challenges with determination. Nancy's younger brother resented the attention that Nancy needed in order to meet the challenges presented by her physical disabilities.

Nancy was born with some hearing loss into a family of people none of whom had any hearing loss. She grew up in what she described as "that in between world" where she was never really accepted as a hearing person, nor was she allowed "membership," as she called it, in the Deaf world. As time and her osteopetrosis gradually robbed her of her hearing and sight, her sign language skills improved and she increasingly was accepted in all three "worlds."

Her childhood was difficult in many ways. With an IQ in the gifted range, she knew that she would want to pursue college studies. However, the barriers to accessibility were often discouraging. Her father did not help her exercise her rights to access services and education. Private schools, despite their more liberal attitudes toward accepting people with differences and special needs, were often the least equipped to provide accessible classrooms and education. Forced to rely on the public school system, Nancy got the best education she could. She eventually attended college and completed her undergraduate degree by the age of 30.

She spent a number of years deciding what she wanted to do next. Her first marriage failed quickly after the initial blush of romance wore off. Her first husband was a hearing person with no physical challenges or disabilities; he had all the vocabulary to be considered a "liberal" on all the right issues, but no patience with Nancy's lifelong, daily needs. She told me that her anger and his fake liberal attitudes were a deadly combination for the marriage.

Meeting her current husband was the start of "the second half of life," as she put it. He also used a wheelchair, had changed his birth name as part of an act of empowerment, and was deeply involved in lobbying and advocacy activities. They supported each other in life and in their work. Although not all was as smooth as it might be, they were deeply committed to each other.

Currently, Nancy was finding herself growing more anxious and depressed about the lack of progress of the disability rights movement in this country. Not knowing how her body might "betray" her next, she felt an urgency to make a difference in the world before she left it behind to "go on to whatever was next in the next life." She impressed me in this interview as a powerful person who was a rich historian of her own life, portraying her successes and failures with pathos, humor, and the gift of a storyteller.

So here we were. The ADA was still a dream for the future. She had issues for counseling that involved the mind, the body, and the spirit. Her social network was a complicated matrix of people with deafness, hearing impairment, and physical disabilities and those who had no disabilities. She had friends in Kansas whom she had left behind and sorely missed, but with whom she kept in touch by TDD. However, this was a challenge in itself because of the lengthy and expensive nature of such long-distance phone relationships. This third session ended with an agreement to meet two to four times per month for a 2-hour block of time to help her cope with the emotional issues of daily life. She was quite clear that the work was to focus on existential here-and-now issues and to stay away from "family of origin crap."

~

The fourth session continued the themes of the third and took us deeper into the pain and humiliation she had suffered at the hands of a culture that discriminated against her, overtly and covertly, by placing barriers to her physical access to services and her access to communication.

Raised by hearing parents in a hearing world, Nancy struggled with the idea that she actually belonged to a different group of people who were hearing impaired. As time went along and her hearing deteriorated, she became more a part of the Deaf community in Kansas. It became a lifelong dream to come to Washington, D.C., and be a part of the hearing-impaired and deaf communities. She wanted to make a difference in the world for people with multiple challenges and disabilities.

She wanted to be sure that I really understood her context and went into detail, risking repeating material from the last session. She explained that, as it pertains to hearing and communication, all people grow up as members of one of three communities: deaf, hearing-impaired, or hearing. Some people are members of two of the three. For example, a hearing child raised by deaf parents becomes bilingual at a very early age and quite aware of the issues of both cultures. However, hearing-impaired people who learn sign language (either ASL or any of the versions of signed English) and who have enough hearing to communicate with hearing people without the use of sign language sometimes talk about belonging neither to the deaf community or the hearing community. Sometimes this is a personal issue relating to personality factors, but most often it is a reality of not really being accepted as part of either community.

Nancy Rainbow was the first person I had ever worked with who had actually experienced being a part of all three communities. As the osteopetrosis systematically robbed her of her hearing, she began to rely almost exclusively on lipreading and sign language. She mostly stopped wearing her hearing aids and became more accepted as a member of the deaf community.

While her initial training had been in Signed Exact English (SEE), she quickly realized that ASL was the language of the future and switched over to using ASL exclusively, unless she was communicating with someone who could only understand SEE. The ASL versus SEE controversy was a passionate one for members of her Deaf community in the late 1970s because SEE was seen as a tool of the dominant hearing culture to impose its own syntax and values on the Deaf communities in this country. Although she grew up with enough hearing to easily learn English syntax and idioms, especially when her hearing aids were of some value to her, she actually preferred the beauty of ASL. She explained that the emergence of ASL as the dominant language for deaf people was akin to the battle decades earlier to overcome the "oralism" movement in schools for the deaf, which attempted to forbid the use of sign language in favor of teaching deaf children to lipread and speak English. We ended the fourth session with a decision to use TC, mixing ASL with spoken English, which I heard and she mostly lipread. It was a delicate dance of communicating simultaneously in two languages, one with the voice and the other with the rest of the body.

Finally, in the fifth session, Nancy felt that I was ready to begin hearing about her current angst regarding life issues. The first major issue she wanted to work on was a great mystery to her. She stated, almost apologetically, that it had relatively nothing to do with deafness, physical challenges, or other painful aspects of her life. She wanted to discuss the anger she felt toward a neighbor who was upset about her cats visiting his yard to play in his garden. She said it was a little enough matter, but she had difficulty getting this man to understand that the cats were litter box trained, did not eat plants, and would not harm his garden. He acknowledged all of this to be true, but stated that he "was a dog person" and never really understood cats. She calmly described to me in a mechanical, almost bored tone that she thought that he was a man of very limited insight and imagination, kind of like her alcoholic father, and that she found his dismissal of her cats to cause unexplainable rage fantasies in her. Although she would never follow through on these images, she took some pains to describe what she thought God might have in store for this man in some circle of hell after his death. Nancy was obviously dealing with some important issues that had surfaced in this seemingly mundane concern regarding her cats. Because we had agreed, however, that my role was to be a supportive counselor, and not a therapist, I refrained from interpreting or probing the meaning of her relationship to her cats. I also avoided the obvious comparisons between her neighbor and her father.

We proceeded through this session, spending what felt like a long time on this issue of the cats, and only resolved that some people have the same bigotry toward cats that they have toward people who are somehow different than themselves. This seemed like a "good enough" use of our time and seemed to assure her that I had no agenda for controlling the course of her counseling. As it turned out, this was exceptionally fortunate, because "control issues" were major factors in the later work we did together.

The sixth session was quite different. It was as if Nancy had recognized on some level of awareness that I was to be trusted with some of her deeper secrets. She wanted to explore the depths of her anxiety and depression in a way that almost overwhelmed me given the mundane focus of our prior session. She did talk of family of origin issues and the impact they had on the here-and-now issues of daily life. We worked on the relationship between her physical challenges and her successes. She connected these themes to her emotional challenges and promised herself she would succeed in the same way. The session went into "double overtime" and left us both drained, but feeling as though the work had taken a new turn that would be productive.

~

The next six sessions occurred over the space of 3 months. For a variety of reasons, including her busy schedule and some cancellations due to bouts of poor health during the colds and flu season, we met an average of twice a month. While this is not my usual preference, it was clearly the best we could do.

She continued to work on here-and-now, there-and-then, and looking-to-the-future issues. The most difficult issues during this phase involved whether to consider her hearing loss as a "disability" or a "challenge." Because she had grown up in the hearing world, and gradually made transitions into being with people who were hearing impaired and deaf, she was quite confused on this issue. She very much agreed with those who were strongly of the opinion that having pride about Deaf culture and language was an empowering position. She had felt the barriers of inaccessibility when interpreters were not provided at large public events she attended, or when her best efforts to arrange for an interpreter were met with funding problems. At the same time, she sometimes felt like an outsider because her hearing loss had come on slowly and progressively over her lifetime; few people she met had had the same experience. In this aspect, the hearing loss felt like a disability similar to her progressive loss of vision. People with limited sight or who were sightless did not have their own language or cultural identity, and most relied on characterizing their limited eyesight as a disability in order to receive needed services from government agencies. This issue was a "hot" one in the Deaf communities of which she was and had been a part.

Finally the relationship issues with her husband surfaced. He was clearly a loving and supportive man. He helped Nancy with many physical tasks. They gave each other emotional support in facing the rigors of daily life. However, like any two people who spend lots of time together, they sometimes irritated each other. I was not trained, at that time, in couples therapy; and they were not interested in doing couples-focused work. But it did seem to help her that she could vent some emotion about minor problems in her marriage in a context where she felt safe that the substance of her venting would remain confidential.

One of the most amazing events in our work happened when Nancy asked me to be an interpreter for her at a disability rights support group that was meeting in her home for 8 hours one Saturday. Here I had the chance to perform a very different function as a support to Nancy. The support group was powerful, and Nancy was the convener. She spoke with authority and pride about her successes and challenges. She communicated deep emotion about her failures and struggles. She was a tremendous support to others in the group, each of whom had different physical challenges and emotional issues. The day flew by, and it changed the course of the work that Nancy and I were doing.

In future sessions, my unconscious prejudices about working with people with disabilities underwent a shift. I made these prejudices a part of the work in order to keep them from remaining unconscious and toxic. We noticed that more "got done" in each session. Nancy shifted her own position to a more powerful one, and we agreed that our time for working together was probably coming to a close over the next months. She felt as though I had done much for her and that it was soon time to move on to whatever was next in her growth.

She decided to purchase a magnifying glass for her TDD readout display. This obviated the need for her husband to assist her in reading telephone conversations. She became increasingly active with the support group and began attending weekend workshops to work through emotional issues in an intensive manner.

~

Termination was natural and easy. We both felt it coming as Nancy grew in spirit, power, and energy. Only occasionally did she fall into the pit of despair that had characterized the worst of her depression. Although she experienced anxiety at times, it did not reach levels beyond that with which she could cope.

Several months after our last session, I was surprised to hear from Nancy that they were moving back to Kansas. Family and friends there missed them too much. They felt like they had done important advocacy work toward passing the ADA, which they believed would some day make a difference in the world. We said our final farewell the way we had met . . . via the TDD.

Some time later, a colleague asked me to address the annual meeting of the Association of Independent Schools of Greater Washington. The topic I selected was "Deaf Cultural Awareness in our Hearing School," which described the language program at the Sandy Spring Friends Middle School. The speech was a plea for schools to reach beyond the walls of their own communities to better understand people with all kinds of differences. In fact, the language program in ASL at the SSF Middle School was a model for involving hearing people in an authentic way with the language, the humor, and the culture of people with hearing problems. It involved our students in exchange programs and athletic competitions with students from the Model Secondary School for the Deaf in Washington, D.C. Unlike students from other hearing schools with whom the MSSD students competed, our students dared to use their rudimentary ASL skills to communicate. They risked the same embarrassment and feelings of language deficiency I had felt keenly in my work with Nancy Rainbow. What a great gift of learning it was to know, even if for just a Saturday morning, what it was like to struggle to be understood. We were treated with admiration by the MSSD students for our willingness to be awkward and to do our best to communicate. Little did these students know how much they owed to Nancy Rainbow, her advocacy and outreach efforts, and her nearly tireless spirit.

13

More Than One Life Story in a Life

Working with Disability Across Cultures

Richard Ruth

An odd contradiction suffuses the intersection between disability and culture. On the one hand, certain aspects of disability seem to rise above culture, to be more independent of culture than many other elements of psychological life: a missing leg is a missing leg, deafness is deafness (giving rise to the misconception that deaf people from all over the world share a common sign language). Yet at the same time, the experience of disability is profoundly culturally mediated. It is as if, stripped of some of our customary beliefs, defenses, and elements of individual autonomy and self-determination by the demands of disability, what is left is a closer connection with the substrate of culture.

This mechanism may underlie some of the ubiquitous stereotyping and conservatizing of people with disabilities (including by people with disabilities ourselves). We cannot conceive of the actual lusts, night dreams, and eccentricities—the full psychological aliveness—of a person with a disability. Therefore we construct people with disabilities as inexorably sweet and patient and split off the awareness that they can be intolerably demanding, self-centered, and cranky. We see them as prototypical Midwesterners, or African Americans, or Chinese. Reductionism of this sort is not entirely illogical or unfair. People with

I am indebted to Mindel Shore, LCSW, for helping to shape my thinking about this case, and to Steve Goldstein, Ph.D., for thoughtful comments on an earlier version of this chapter.

disabilities often have the experience that we have limited space for the development of our own personal uniqueness and that we have to rely on and conform to the culture in which we live more than we might like. Nevertheless, it is important to identify what is distorted and what is objective, how the various decisions and compromises feel, what is a choice and what is an imposition in these cases. This complex and treacherous task is integral to effective therapy and lies at its core.

~

Patients tell us their stories in different ways. Some do so directly, in clearly organized narratives. Others speak in false narratives, and the struggle then is to extract the truth. Still others tell their stories in even less direct ways—by their bearing and tone, by what they do not or cannot say, or perhaps by enactment, by what they show more than by what they say.

A challenge of cross-cultural therapy is the need to take a stance that is both neutral and attuned. We need to attend to what patients tell us, but also to *how* they describe their experiences and feelings, and think carefully about what subtleties of tone and word choice may mean. Our interventions need to be attuned and responsive to these subtleties of nuance if we are to be truly helpful.

This leads to something very disquieting: We can never understand the material of a patient from another culture as well as the material of a patient from our own culture, and yet we have to help patients develop a deep, culturally rooted understanding of what they tell us nevertheless. If we can go even further and talk with our patients about what we do not understand, why there is confusion, what our confusion feels like, and what meanings this might imply, then cross-cultural therapy can become truly exciting and productive.

~

I want to start the story of my work with don Rogelio in the middle, with an incident that occurred about a year and a half into my work with him. We were talking about some difficulty he had been having, over a period of several weeks, understanding what was entailed in applying for Social Security disability benefits. Yet again, I had explained some of the process to him, and he had nodded his agreement and made comments suggesting he understood; soon after, however, he said something indicating he had a completely erroneous idea of what was involved.

I mentioned this to him and wondered aloud what this behavior meant. Don Rogelio startled me by saying that for the duration of our time together he had had trouble understanding me, that I spoke unclearly and that often he had no idea what I was saying.

Don Rogelio and I both share a connection to Latin American culture, and the therapy was conducted entirely in Spanish. However, we are rooted in very different parts of Latin America and our accents and usage patterns differ. We are also from different economic and educational backgrounds, and our life stories differ radically. I have been in the United States longer than he; I speak English, he does not. In fact, from time to time we both had trouble understanding each other's speech and language, although we had never discussed it. But as we explored don Rogelio's comment and used it as a springboard to reflect together for the first time on the course of our therapeutic work, we made some startling discoveries. Primarily, we determined that there were very basic things we did not understand about each other and the sustained conversation in which we were engaged. Fortunately, though, we had a sufficient basis of trust and mutual concern that it was now possible to think about it, talk about it, and explore its potential mysteries and meanings.

There are at least two versions of don Rogelio's history. I would like to recount these and then speculate about the meaning and implications of the differences.

Don Rogelio was originally referred to me by a private rehabilitation firm. He had worked as a painter and had an accident at work, where he fell off a ladder and broke his feet. The rehabilitation nurse managing the case, a capable and compassionate woman from my native country, felt that don Rogelio was basically a bright and psychologically competent man who was experiencing some anxiety and depression related to his injuries and the long recovery from them. This was interfering with his imminent return to work. She wanted me to see him for focal therapy, and I agreed.

When I took an initial history from don Rogelio, he denied any peculiar early life circumstances or any psychological difficulties prior to the accident, except that he used to drink but had not had a drinking problem for several years. But when don Rogelio first came into my office, he was clearly in considerable pain. It is always hard to tell what is somatic and what is of psychological etiology in a person with chronic pain. In an attempt to sort this out, I asked don Rogelio about his accident in an open-ended way.

He told me he had lost his footing on a ladder, half-smiling in the way men uncomfortable talking about their feelings often do. He talked about it the way a good soccer player may talk ruefully about missing a goal he should have gotten. But, he asked me, why did I think it was that his back as well as his feet hurt so much all the time?

I soon learned that after the accident don Rogelio was taken to a local hospital, where an orthopedic surgeon did emergency surgery, and over the following months several follow-up surgeries, on his feet, which were now held together by a series of pins and wires. However, the doctor did not speak Spanish, and he breezed in and out quickly. When I phoned the doctor and mentioned the back pain, he told me rather arrogantly that the problem was the broken feet, that feet were what he dealt with, and that I was a psychologist and should deal with the psychology. I suppressed my feelings and asked him if he had ever examined don Rogelio's back. When he told me he had not and did not intend to, I soon found myself telling him that if he did not examine and X-ray don Rogelio's back, I would pursue the matter at whatever level necessary. He took the X-ray, and it was then discovered don Rogelio had been walking around for a year and a half with two fractured vertebrae. The doctor grudgingly approved a course of physical therapy, which was of some help but was inadequte to relieve the pain.

I remember thinking, after my moment of crisis about whether I had lost my ability to communicate in Spanish, that don Rogelio must have understood something of what I had been saying to him if we had negotiated such a powerful episode together. And, indeed, the work around the quality of his medical care had opened up a number of issues. In fact, what caused the fall was not a slip in don Rogelio's macho footing. Rather, the contractor for whom he was working had disarmed a safety device on the ladder so it would go a few feet higher and the company would not have to buy a more expensive ladder. This made the ladder sufficiently unstable that don Rogelio fell. The hard realization that construction contractors almost routinely do such things to local Latino workers, and to other construction workers across the country, was overwhelming to both of us. Our ability to contain and metabolize such an enraging and saddening realization is at the heart of the empathic connection that drove the first period of the therapy.

Further, don Rogelio's inability to be assertive with his medical doctor was an important finding. He was unable to express directly to the doctor the rage about him that he expressed to me; indeed, at times he communicated the diametrical opposite to the doctor. This was a profound phenomenon, both cultural and psychological, which we discussed at length. When the doctor began an appointment with don Rogelio, he would begin by asking him how he was. Don Rogelio, as a polite Central American, would answer that he was fine, thank you, and inquire about the doctor and his family, with the expectation that, with this polite greeting ritual negotiated, the doctor would then start telling stories, examine him carefully, offer him coffee, and, after enough time, let don Rogelio tell him how he really felt—the rituals of medical care in Central America. When, instead, the doctor would brusquely write down that don Rogelio said he was fine and leave the room, don Rogelio was dumbfounded and too humiliated to say anything. He revealed these feelings only to me, in this odd extended conversation we were having.

I had moments of doubt and conflict about approaching a medical colleague so confrontationally. Was I disempowering don Rogelio by not insisting he deal with this problem himself? Was I going beyond what don Rogelio could tolerate? Was I inappropriately projecting my own rage onto don Rogelio, thus sabotaging the therapy by acting out a countertransference (i.e., my unconscious feelings evoked by his unconscious feelings toward me)? Would the story get around, cutting me off from referral sources and branding me as a dangerous extremist in the professional community? Or, was this a moment where my willingness to fight hard for what was right could open up new possibilities in therapy? If so, how would I harness and communicate this potential to don Rogelio? Even reflecting in retrospect, I do not know the answer to these questions.

I concluded that there was nothing acceptable about allowing a patient of mine to walk around with a broken back; an inner voice was telling me insistently that this was the moment for action. Sometimes action at a pivotal point in the development of a therapy brings along rich insight, cultural and psychological, that is not possible at earlier or later points in the process. So, metaphorically, I willingly jumped off the cliff.

~

Clearly, this had not been a therapy where patient and therapist were disconnected or where little happened. But don Rogelio told me a different version of his story after we talked about his difficulty understanding me. The new rendition went like this:

Don Rogelio is the second youngest of seven children. His family is from a rural zone of El Salvador, one known for the unusual abundance and beauty of its land. The family owned a considerable amount of land and lived a life that was considered quite advantaged in Salvadorean terms. This does not translate easily into an urban, North American frame of reference. For example, this "rich" family lived without electricity, farm machinery, or much in the way of formal education. Don Rogelio recalls his earliest years in Arcadian terms and tells great stories about managing the family's oxen and knocking ripe mangoes out of a tree with a stick.

When don Rogelio was 5 years old, his father died. His death resulted from a combination of the chronic health deficits related to the intensely hard work of the underdeveloped Third World and an acute infection from poor sanitary conditions in the Salvadorean countryside. His mother, whom he describes as a weak woman, was easily overwhelmed and left the running of the family's lands to don Rogelio's older male siblings. They could not effectively manage the agricultural undertaking, so that soon much of the land was sold or mortgaged, and the yields were no longer abundant on the remaining cultivated lands and on the animals they raised. The brothers drank and ran around in a nearby town. They treated don Rogelio abusively. They would beat him, burden him with onerous duties, insult him, and berate him verbally to the point of nightly tears. They took him out of school after the second grade so he could work longer hours and sometimes denied him food.

When he was 8, don Rogelio left home. He worked on rubber and coffee plantations as a migrant laborer for the next 4 years, often working for food rather than wages. What wages he did earn he gave mostly to his mother. He began drinking to ease his loneliness, hunger, and physical and emotional pain.

When he was 12, don Rogelio moved to San Salvador, his country's capital, where he lived on the streets for the next 4 years. He drank heavily, worked irregularly, and had a marginal existence. One day when he was 16, he was with a bunch of street urchins begging from passersby in a nice part of town. Something about his assertive repartee caught the attention of a passerby, who happened to be a clinical psychologist. The psychologist invited him for a meal, and they spoke at length. The psychologist invited don Rogelio to move into his home and do household work for him.

This arrangement lasted for the next 9 months. Don Rogelio was a good worker and had a kindness and a brightness that endeared him to the psychologist, who got him medical care, fed and clothed him properly, and tried to get him into school. But don Rogelio could make no progress in school, in spite of his best efforts and the psychologist's nightly assistance. They discussed this together, and the psychologist suggested that don Rogelio had little future in his country, by then enveloped in war and a collapsing economy. The psychologist arranged for him to come, illegally, to the United States. Don Rogelio traveled on foot through Mexico to the Texas border, crossed with the help of a *coyote* (someone who helps Latinos cross the border into the United States illegally), and made his way to California. There he lived in overcrowded apartments with other single men, drank heavily, and worked for minimum wage in factories.

This lasted until he met his wife, a widow with children. They fell in love, the drinking eased up a bit, and they moved to the Washington, D.C., area. Here, don Rogelio's natural intelligence and capacity for hard work led him to become an increasingly skilled construction worker and then a painter. He was drinking episodically, working regularly, and making almost $20 an hour when he had his accident. This was the "uneventful life" he had initially told me about.

I was speechless after hearing this revised story, the more so when don Rogelio told me that, in fact, he had known me before we began therapy. It turned out I had tested his oldest stepdaughter for the local schools 2 years before I began seeing him for therapy. The daughter has moderate mental retardation, and I recalled her as a delightful and well-adjusted young woman whom I had seen for a routine school evaluation. Don Rogelio had retreated to a recliner in the den after greeting me politely, while I spoke, by his request, to his wife about the findings.

Whole worlds linger under seemingly routine surfaces. Sometimes, if we are lucky and skillful and have sufficient space and time, we can learn about them in long-term therapy. After don Rogelio told me this version of his life story, it began to make sense to me why his recovery from the accident had been so long and uneven. The accident layered over earlier trauma and restimulated it, constraining don Rogelio's availability for the physical and psychological work of recovery. I marveled at how much don Rogelio had been able to cross the barriers of culture, disability, class, and dialect to finally tell me this deeper story. And I wondered how on earth I could really help him, at the same time realizing that his entrusting me with his story was an act rich with therapeutic potential.

What has worked in our therapy, now continuing into its fourth year? Paradoxically, we have done very little not prescribed in classic thinking about technique. We meet regularly, with careful attention to starting and ending on time and to other basic ground rules. Don Rogelio has been encouraged to talk about anything. I will most often say very little, but my occasional questions and interpretations are oriented toward trying to help him understand the meanings and implications of his thoughts and feelings and their flow or restriction. Sometimes we talk about dreams and what *they* mean. Don Rogelio has had the experience that sometimes my comments hit the mark. He may retrieve a memory or see an experience in a new way; sometimes it is healing for him to share, release, or find words for a complex emotion. I model talking openly and without shame about disability issues. At the same time, don Rogelio knows that if he asks me a direct informational question—about how Social Security works, or a problem his daughter is having in school, for example—I am not incapable of giving him a direct answer. In other words, I do not hesitate to weave a psychoeducational element into the flow of therapy, if I believe it will be helpful.

One way culture makes a difference in don Rogelio's case is that such long-term, in-depth therapy is rare in Salvadorean culture for people with don Rogelio's disabilities. There are other culturally driven differences as well. We speak in Spanish and use some of the conventions common to those elements of our cultures that have a common Hispanic root. I will ask him politely about his family by way of greeting, and not just about him as an individual, as I might with a North American patient. When at the end of a session I say I will see him the following week, his culturally normative response is *si dios quiere*—"if God wills it"; that is, in the gentle tone of a common refrain, I should know better than to think that we humans are ever enough in control of things that we can really predict what will happen from week to week. I am not sure what the therapy would be like, or if it would work at all, if there were not this subtle measure of shared cultural experience, or if I did not have an empathic sense about what it is like to live with disability and pain.

There are more profound cultural phenomena that enter the therapy as well. Don Rogelio's subjective sense of time is primarily cyclical rather than clock time. He has a deeply founded belief that most of life is fated and that the operative range of free will is much less than most North Americans would presume. He has a sense that multiple narratives can coexist. Thus, his presentation of two radically different versions of his life is not something he sees as a flow from defense to openness. Rather, it is rooted in a deep belief that there is more than one way of understanding the world and oneself and that, at different times and in different contexts and affective climates, one or the other becomes more overt or prominent. Sometimes he can walk well and does not feel disabled; sometimes he can barely move, does not get a decent night's sleep for days and weeks, and is in constant pain.

Much of psychotherapy and the thinking about disability of most people in this society is based on the assumption that people have a great deal of control over what happens to them and that history is more objective than subjective. Therapists often find that we gain tremendous leverage for change by challenging scripts—that is, by helping people see their life histories and experience their disabilities with different explanatory perspectives. The whole therapeutic enterprise becomes decentered when people live comfortably with multiple, not necessarily mutually complementary explanations of their experience, as don Rogelio does. Perhaps we should be open to moments with all patients when this radical shift in world view seems possible.

I do not make interpretations about these elements to don Rogelio, just as I would not comment in a text upon the ways that cultural thinking affects my writing. Perhaps it is enough simply to describe the subjective experience of a person with a disability from a culture other than the dominant one in the United States. When this kind of experience is appreciated from a position of empathic understanding, the implications can be so radical that it is hard to grasp them directly. The relevant points need to be gotten across gently and indirectly.

As best as I can understand, the culturally related phenomena I have tried to describe in this case study constitute one important layer of the contents of therapy. Awareness, not interpretation, of them bolsters my ability to be an effective empathic containing vessel, the single most essential ingredient for a therapy like this to progress.

14

Sally

Recovery of Our Missing Pieces

Karen Donovan

It is essential that we give voice to the experience of having physical disabilities in this society. How those of us with disabilities from early childhood attempt to heal ourselves is an issue of great importance. Some would argue that focusing on the wounds of people with disabilities promotes them as victims needing charity and deserving pity, and suggests that they have serious problems to overcome. I don't agree. We have been silent too long and our silence has hurt us psychologically as well as socially and politically. The recent emphasis on accessibility barriers, both architectural and attitudinal, has been helpful in promoting the view of people with disabilities as a minority group in need of its own civil rights. At the same time, it has made us more conscious of how much the disability experience has directly affected our own sense of who we are, how we relate to others, and how we view the world. Exploration of these areas can only help to recover missing pieces of ourselves—pieces that were locked out of awareness and denied expression because of the demands and standards of the external world that forced us to construct a sense of self that was not genuine.

Freud claimed that the self-representation (the total way we see ourselves) is first and foremost a body representation. Initially, the child is able to take in only crude representations of pleasure and unpleasure through need-satisfying activities like being fed. Gradually he begins to distinguish self from other and perceives sensations arising from various sources. He organizes and structures them in such a way that representations are formed of both self and other (Sandler &

Rosenblatt, 1962, p. 131). It is through the body, then, that the child first experiences who he is in relationship to the mother or caretaker and the world. Jacobson (1964) writes that the child's earliest experiences of pleasure and unpleasure or gratification and frustration "constitute the first and most significant bridge to the mother" (p. 35). As these earliest experiences of the child of being gratified and frustrated accrue, they form images of the mother which they in turn take in as their first self-image or self-representation. It is easy to see that a disability might alter the mother's interaction with her child and consequently affect the child's emerging sense of self. For example, the mother of a child with a physical disability might not be able to provide enough of these early pleasurable experiences. She may not be able or know how to respond to the cues given out by the baby that would enable him or her to feel safe, and at one with the world. The mother's uncomfortable, scared, or pained attitude and behavior may cause the child to feel excessively frustrated, and the excessively frustrated child cannot develop a sense of cohesion.

In describing the earliest infant–mother interactions, Winnicott (1982) says that what the baby sees when he looks into the mother's face reflects what the mother sees while she is looking at her baby. If the mother does not reflect back what she sees but what she wants to see, the child does not develop a sense of himself that is real, but one that is false (p. 118). Thus, it is important that the child find himself, his own true nature, reflected in the mother's look and not her own troubled mood or own image of who he should be instead of who he is. A mother who confronts the reality of her child with a disability has to deal with her own sense of wholeness. The subsequent anxieties about her own competency as a mother and caregiver, both physical and psychological, are reflected in her interactions with her infant. If the anxieties are too great or the frustration too excessive, the child will have a difficult time forming a sense of self that is cohesive, stable, and genuine.

Many people with disability whom I have seen in therapy have expressed feelings of having to wear a mask to the world. The mask reflects what the world wants to see, not the true self. The true or real self, never having been reflected or mirrored back, is lost. Recovering these missing pieces of ourselves can sometimes be arduous and time consuming. What follows is the story of Sally and her journey to find her own self, to exist, and to feel real. My work was to do what had not been done before, to be there and reflect back what she brought me. As the skin horse in the Velveteen Rabbit affirms, *real* is not about how you are made, but rather is something that happens to you . . . It is what happens when someone loves you (Williams, 1984).

~

Sally was born prematurely, weighing a little less than 2 pounds. Survival at that weight in the early 1950s was rare. Her parents were told that, should she live, she would be so incapacitated that they should consider institutionalization. She remained in the hospital for several months, during which time only her father came to see her. Her mother's absence from the hospital has never been adequately understood. All developmental milestones were delayed; for example, she did not start walking until she was nearly 5. She was diagnosed as having cerebral palsy.

What became clear as her story unfolded was that her parents, particularly her mother, had a great deal of emotional difficulty with the disability. From the beginning, it seems the goal was for Sally to overcome her disability or at least diminish the external appearance of disability as much as possible. It is interesting that when the disability was finally acknowledged it was done in a way that felt very exploitative to Sally. Sally endured many surgical procedures and endless physical therapy to improve and correct her walking. She was constantly reminded to make adjustments to the way she walked or held her hands or in her facial expressions.

She had no affiliation with any agency that dealt with disability. She was told she wasn't like them. The minimizing and even denial of her limitations often resulted in Sally having to navigate physical situations that were nearly overwhelming for her. For example, there were stairs with no railing in both her home and school. Sally was mainstreamed from the beginning. She neither knew nor saw any other children with disabilities except when she visited the hospital. Her first years in school were very difficult. She was often laughed at, had no friends, and did poorly academically. Interestingly, several years into her schooling it was discovered that she had a serious visual problem and prescription glasses turned her academic work around. From then on, she was an above-average student, getting honors in high school.

Sally's childhood was spent trying to overcome her differentness, a differentness that was apparently intolerable for her parents. She alternated between being fearful of not being able to meet her parents' expectations and being rageful and depressed at all the demands being placed on her. There seems to have been little joy. She was a project to be worked on and made whole. Sally often says, "My mother was obsessed with me." There was an expectation, verbalized or not, that she would one day not have a disability, that all her efforts would one day be rewarded, and she could then enjoy life and have the kind of life she saw others having. Sally clearly had little sense of control in her life. Her mother chose her clothes, her friends, and her food and demanded the highest standards of behavior from her. She feared her mother's look of disapproval and anger. When Sally reached her own limit with all of these demands, she would refuse to do anything but sit and read or watch TV, sometimes for weeks at a time.

It could be said that Sally was given two conflicting messages from her mother: "You need me to function in this world" and "You will achieve great things if you work hard and overcome your disability." When Sally was 10 her mother became ill. She stepped up her efforts to please her mother even more, working harder and spending more time with her. She died when Sally was in her last year of high school. The last thing Sally recalls her mother saying before she died concerned the way she was walking. She reports that, after her mother's death, her father went into a deep depression and became emotionally unavailable.

Sally was able to secure the financial and emotional help she needed to go on to college. After she graduated she was rejected for numerous jobs, but she finally landed a job that assured her financial security and seemed to be within her physical capabilities. After several years, however, she began to experience extreme exhaustion. She found the work too demanding and felt overwhelmed all the time. She began a continuous struggle with increasing illness and depression and was absent from work a great deal. Finally, she was forced to reduce her hours considerably so that she could no longer financially make it on her own. Initially, she refused any help in getting subsidized housing, supplemental disability income, or medical benefits. To accept them would mean she had failed. When it became clear that she had to have help to survive, she reluctantly gave in.

Sally came to my office having been referred by the local independent living center. In our first meeting together, I recall how pressured I felt by her. Her words gushed out. She was overwhelmed with sadness and cried throughout the session. She was riddled with anxiety and was in jeopardy of losing her apartment and her job. She was in a crisis, overwhelmed and exhausted, but she had little compassion or empathy for herself. Halfway through the session I realized she did not see herself as having any significant physical limitations. She blamed herself for being a failure.

Sally expressed herself well and demonstrated a certain amount of psychological insight. She appeared to have minimal disabilities—a somewhat unsteady gait was all that was visible. I recall feeling tired and moved by her all at once. I believed that because I have a disability I might more easily be able to help her explore her own experiences with disability. I had polio as a child and have a visible disability. She recalls to this day how good it felt to her when in that first session I validated how much she had already accomplished. She experienced people as always expecting more from her than she could give. She blamed it on the fact that she, unlike me, did not have an obvious disability. However, the reality is that people with disabilities often speak of the need of those without disabilities to either minimize or deny their limitations or to exaggerate their incapacitation. It is a way to handle the strong anxieties about loss, vulnerability, and weakness that get stirred up when they are confronted by a person with a disability. In either case, the person with a disability is denied the experience of being seen for who he or she is.

In our work together those first few months, Sally struggled to understand what had happened to her. She questioned whether she could have or should be doing more, if she was truly ill or if it was her depression that made it so difficult for her to do good things for herself. Other times she blamed others for not giving her enough support, validation, or understanding. We continue to work on these themes. At first it was clear that my nonjudgmental, empathic style caused her a great deal of anxiety. She asked if this was a new kind of therapy: "You understand so much and don't tell me what I should be doing or feeling. My other therapist [who did not have a disability] used to tell me that I should be doing more and threatened to stop seeing me if I didn't shape up. This doesn't feel real that you're being so nice to me."

She obsessively focused on events in her childhood that had been particularly traumatic but which she had never before allowed herself to think about as hurtful or injurious. As the memories and feelings flooded into her consciousness, it often seemed that she was truly reexperiencing her past. Her feelings overwhelmed her. She would ask if what she was remembering had really happened: "Am I making this up? I didn't know all these feelings were here. Why am I remembering my mom only in all negative ways? I know there were good things, but I'm not remembering them right now." Clearly she disassociated the cumulative trauma associated with her disability. I was able to help her understand that her feelings, which seemed to be dangerous and destructive, were actually what she had mirrored by looking into her mother's eyes. It was her mother who was afraid of her own feelings toward her child, and Sally had learned from her.

At first, her angry feelings were intolerable to her. She would allow them in for seconds and then immediately defend against them with intellectualization. I realized that she, like her mother, felt her anger unbearable. Frequently anger permeated the room. I often found myself stuck with the anger that was so difficult for her to accept. Other times I felt angry at her for staying in the past and not getting on with her life. It is easy to become frightened and run away from intense feelings, but it was essential that I stay with her painful feelings to help her recover the lost split-off parts of her that were contained in her early childhood memories and affects. As we went on this journey together, she gained a broadening awareness of what she needed and did not get from her environment. My ability to listen and feel would eventually lead to her being able to listen and feel empathically to her internal world. She needed to separate out that which was hers and that which was her mother's and form her own separate identity. Sally had totally identified with her mother. She needed to separate and mourn.

As Sally's feelings became more tolerable to her, she began ever so slowly to use me as someone who could help her. Her continued exposure to the independent living center staff (most of which were people with disabilities) and clients had an effect on her. At first, she spent many sessions sharing with me how uncomfortable she felt with such people, realizing then that, of course, she held her self in such contempt. Slowly she looked at her own belief system that defined disability in such a devalued way. She questioned the values and standards that had been hers and began to see what a disservice they had done to her. Her anger, still a difficult emotion for her, took on a different quality. It became more consistently focused outward, shifting the locus of control out to society. Perhaps the response was not entirely appropriate, but it was certainly more tolerable and became the motivating force for growth both internally and externally. I find that with many people first discovering their disability from a sociological/political perspective, there is a sense of relief as they feel the blame lifting from themselves onto other more malign forces. Initially it may represent a trying on of values and beliefs that are not yet their own but that provide the opportunity to be part of a community, to belong, to feel a part of something that offers a sense of pride—a totally new feeling.

Sally joined an advocacy group and began to do more volunteer work. She had by this time completely left her job. She had become increasingly aware of how difficult and unsatisfying the work had been for her. Increasingly she saw herself as someone who had been betrayed by society. In trying to keep up and do it all, she realized that she had accepted the general view that disability was something to be overcome and denied. Within a short period of time others in the group admired her and sought her advice and direction. Soon she was chosen as president of the advocacy group. Of course she struggled with whether she deserved the position, but at the same time she found it rewarding and challenging. She grasped ideas quickly and demonstrated a willingness to learn.

Interestingly, while on the outside she evidenced so much growth in our sessions the depression and sense of worthlessness were never more apparent. The attention she was getting from the disability community had stirred up strong feelings of aggression. She wanted more: more acknowledgment, more accommodation, and more visibility in the disability community. Her mother, she realized, would not have approved of her alliance with people with disabilities. But if she could be the star, the leader, it might be something her mother could tolerate. She returned to feeling a great deal of self-loathing and doubt and began to desert the group. In addition, she frequently missed appointments. We had up to this time been meeting regularly twice a week; suddenly she wanted to come only once a week. She complained of increasing illness and disability related problems. The target of her anger was more and more the agency that had not appreciated her hard work. She felt neglected and disappointed. My attempts to point out that that was how she must have felt with her parents when they did not validate all her efforts were met with tears and affirmation, but further exploration proved impossible.

The grieving returned and she became once again immobilized. Their shortcomings felt like her shortcomings. I realized I had to be cautious and sparing with my interventions for she was quick to see them as criticisms aimed at her. It was clear through the transference that a part of her was seeing me as the critical, disapproving mother. She wanted to both please me and do whatever it was she perceived that I wanted from her (like working harder in her therapy and returning to the group); at the same time she wanted me to leave her alone to do nothing. I understood how important it was that I remain empathic to her struggle and that I not have any expectations for her. She needed to feel safe. As she relaxed more in the transference, our relationship became easier for her to talk about. She discovered that she had great fears of growing dependent upon me. Dependency meant being engulfed, smothered, and controlled. It was terrifying to her. One day she came and announced that she had been asked to speak at a disability-related consumer forum. She was delighted and pleased to be acknowledged. She worked hard and got good feedback. She returned to her advocacy work and began to train others in advocacy skills. She proved to be a good speaker and was asked with more and more frequency to speak on disability issues.

~

Sally had entered therapy torn between conflicting feelings of failure and betrayal. She had done all that had been expected of her, yet she had not reached the goals that had been set for her. She had unknowingly become like her mother, embracing idealized standards that did not include disability. Confronted with the increasing awareness that she did indeed have a disability, she saw herself as a devalued person with no power and status. In part, the goal of the therapy became to help her change those values that defined disability in such negative light. She needed to go back and find out who she was and what was important to her apart from her mother. To do that, she needed to first feel safe enough with me that I would value and respect whatever she gave me that was hers. Once that was established, she could allow herself the freedom to discover her own sense of who she was without fear of judgment (hers as well as mine). She was reordering those values that had been so much a part of her.

Sally's adaptation to her disability now displays greater integration of both positive and negative values. The negative, debilitating self-image has been replaced by a more authentic self-representation that includes pieces of her that she discovered in her journey to a greater understanding of herself.

REFERENCES

Jacobson, E. (1964). *The self and the object world.* New York: International Universities Press.

Sandler, J., & Rosenblatt, B. (1962). *The concept of the representational world. The psychoanalytical study of the child, Vol. XVII.* New York: International Universities Press.

Winnicott, D.W. (1982). *Playing and reality.* London: Tavistock.

Williams, M. (1984). *The velveteen rabbit.* Philadelphia: Courage Books.

15

Sam

In Search of Love

Adele Natter

When I tell people that my work involves psychotherapy with persons with mental retardation, invariably I hear the conventional wisdom, namely, that the task is impossible. How can psychotherapy help someone who is so intellectually impaired? How can someone who has not developed higher cortical functions, whose cognitive development stopped at a very low mental age, benefit from "the talking cure," traditionally the sphere of angst-ridden intellectuals? I believe the answer to this puzzling question is that persons with cognitive impairments—and psychotherapy itself—are capable of more than we tend to suppose. Like many other persons, I used to assume that people with mental retardation live lives of blissful ignorance, that "what they don't know won't hurt them." Sam taught me that this is not the case.

~

During the early period of my professional development, I began to treat clients with developmental disabilities and was assigned to be Sam's therapist. When I read this man's intake summary, I began to have my doubts. The day I actually met Sam, my heart sank. I was wondering to myself what could be done for this man.

The intake process is an attempt at a comprehensive understanding of the potential new client. Background information, such as work or school evaluations, psychological testing, and social summaries, is requested. Then the client is interviewed, often together with his or her parent or counselor, to understand the individual's perspective on his or her life and current problems. We desire to understand what biological, social and psychological forces are interacting with the individual's psyche and how these have come together to propel the person toward psychiatric treatment now. The intake assessment had been done by another therapist. I saw that Sam had been identified as having moderate mental retardation and a diagnosis of organic brain syndrome. Even at his supervised job, which involved doing outdoor maintenance as part of a groundskeeping crew, he would become distracted from his assigned tasks. In addition, his group home counselors had compiled a lengthy list of negative behaviors which, in all probability, had been reinforced by a long history of institutionalization, beginning at the age of 13. He was now 38.

The initial session was no more reassuring. Sam was, by any standard, a mess. His clothes were disheveled: his shirt was untucked, his cuffs had slipped beneath the heels of his shoes, his belt was only half-buckled, and his pants were threatening to fall down his tall, thin figure. A hirsute individual, Sam had a "5 o'clock shadow," even though it was morning. His shirt was stained with food and his sleeve was dirty where he had used it to wipe his mouth. He repeatedly begged his companions to buy him a soda.

A chief complaint about Sam among his counselors concerned his hyperactivity. Sam's behavior in my office was consistent with the reports: he was in constant motion. He sucked his thumb, rubbed his head, talked to himself, and made shrieking noises. He paced the floor like a caged animal. Indeed, the office could barely contain him, and he made numerous announcements that he needed to go to the bathroom.

Unsure how to proceed with the client, I turned my attention to the medical liaison who had accompanied him to the initial interview. It was her job to make appointments for medical and dental services and to transport the clients to those appointments. Wearily, the medical liaison enumerated additional problems that Sam posed to the staff of the group home, which had been his home for the past 3 years: He talked to himself in one voice and answered in another. He made violent threats and got into fights with his housemate (also his friend), Jay. He made inappropriate overtures to members of the opposite sex. Sam was very impulsive. He had a tendency to use abusive language, and there were times when he had run away from home. One time, he jumped off the deck, spraining his ankle.

Another problem for the residential counselors, she said, was keeping Sam presentable. A casual glance verified the truth of this statement. The therapist wrote in the intake evaluation, "Even when he has dressed carefully, he will look disheveled after a short time." When upset, he would tear his clothes off. He rubbed his head when excited, scratched his head when irritated, and sucked his thumb much of the time, out of habit. Like an infant, he put things into his mouth impulsively, and he sometimes took food out of the garbage to eat.

The medical liaison did not come right out and say, "Tell him to stop these behaviors," but it was tacitly understood that that was her agenda, why she had brought Sam to the clinic, and why she was willing to continue bringing him to appointments. The house staff were overburdened and overwhelmed; besides Sam, there were five other men in the group home, four of them nonverbal. I glanced over at him. He hung his head as she recited everything that he had done wrong; he was being humiliated in front of me. He promised he would never do those things again; he wanted to get out of here. He was sure he was in big trouble now and doomed to punishment.

~

I had just met these people, and already I felt I had a conflict. What was my primary task here? Was it to make this anxious client, who was being called to account for his misbehaviors, more comfortable? Was it to make the client stop these nonproductive, uncooperative actions and give the obviously overburdened counselor some relief? I thought about the point at which I should enter this system—the best place to enter the therapy.

I decided that although the counselors had needs—for support, guidance, management techniques, more resources—they also had more internal resources and patience than their client. I needed to teach my new client—and the medical liaison—about the therapeutic process: that here, in this room, we would talk about problems and feelings and that we can do this in a conversational manner. Also, if I could help the client to reduce his anxiety and engage in the treatment, in talking honestly to me, then the medical liaison and counselors would ultimately feel the benefit of this process as well. I planned to talk more with the medical liaison later, when I felt I had a better understanding of what was happening internally to the client. To begin helping Sam, I needed to convince him that he was not here to be judged or punished and that I was in his corner. For myself, to proceed with this work, I needed to find likable qualities in him so that I could care about him and regard him positively.

This positive view from the therapist is itself, I believe, helpful to people who have learned from their interactions with others that their intelligence and behavior are considered substandard. Even speaking of the client's worst behavior, impulses, or thoughts can transform them into understandable events in the context of the client's life and should not change the therapist's positive feelings toward the client. By being valued by the therapist, the client comes to value himself and own those aspects of his nature that the therapist treasures. While it is true that the worker has to address the problems and undesirable behaviors that so disturb those around the client, a substantial part of therapy is recognizing and reinforcing those positive elements that are unique to the person. Therapeutic change takes place through the formation of a supporting and accepting relationship between client and therapist. In this respect and in many others, the process of therapy with a person with mental disabilities is similar to all psychotherapy.

One difference is that, in general, people without disabilities self-refer for treatment because they are uncomfortable with their symptoms or realize that their mood or outlook has changed for the worse. Perhaps they recognize that if they do not change their behavior, negative consequences will ensue. On the other hand, persons with developmental disabilities are often brought to therapy because their problems and undesirable behaviors disturb those around them. The client's social environment responds to this disturbance by bringing the person to therapy to be "fixed." This reflects the behaviorally oriented approach that seems to be prevalent in systems that work with such populations. In my experience, rare is the client with mental retardation who is brought for therapy because he or she seems to be merely unhappy. In fact, the pressures on the residential system are such that if residents are withdrawn or crying in their rooms, for example, as opposed to acting out, nothing will be done about it; their feelings are expressed upon themselves and often are not considered problematic. But if a resident's behavior contributes to a crisis for the household, that resident's behavior gets attention. This, then, was the pressure I was feeling in the initial interview: to convince the medical liaison that treatment would help and that her time and effort to bring Sam would relieve the burdens of caring for him, while simultaneously attempting to convince myself that I would find a way to relate to and care for this grossly unappealing man.

I shared with the medical liaison that this process would take time. It was tempting to relate primarily to the medical liaison, who, after all, is reasonable and caring and more like a peer. I recognized how difficult, embarrassing, and ungratifying it is for the medical liaisons and counselors to work with someone like Sam. I needed their help to understand his deficits in order to work on either "fixing" them or to help his social contacts to accept him as he was. I also suggested that they take Sam and his housemates on more outings into the community, which they did, although not as often as Sam and I would have liked.

~

The medical liaison sometimes served a filtering or brokering function; that is, Sam's behavior of the recent past was reported to the medical liaison, who reported it to me. Conversely, when I involved the medical liaison in the therapy session, or brought her in for a summary of what we were working on, she presumably relayed this information back to the group home staff. One reason I say "presumably" is that there was frequent turnover in the group home staff, a common situation in residential systems for people with mental retardation. For various reasons, including low pay, career changes, illness, failure to get recertified, and jockeying available staff to provide coverage, there were several periods in which the medical liaison was a more stable presence in Sam's life than the group home counselors.

One of my jobs as therapist was to help Sam understand these changes, process these losses of people who were important to him, and help him say goodbye whenever possible. Unfortunately, some of his counselors did not give enough notice to make this closure feasible. At times when the medical liaison position was unfilled, the overnight counselor, who was now working overtime, brought Sam to his morning therapy appointment. One can hardly blame this employee for falling asleep in the waiting room, but he was not able to be an effective liaison, either. Perhaps this lethargy filtered down from the administrator of Sam's group home. She was slow to respond to Sam's requests or my suggestions, especially if they required some work on her part.

One of the first messages I wanted to get across to Sam was that this was a safe place to come and to discuss what was happening; he would not be punished for the things he told me, but we would talk about them. In the beginning of the therapy, Sam would lie to make his actions seem better than they had been and to save face.

Gradually he was able to stay in the office for longer periods before needing to leave to go to the bathroom. On these excursions he was curious about other people, their offices, and the objects in them. He had little sense of appropriate boundaries; if an object attracted his interest, he would ask to keep it. His neediness was apparent to all, and this open and unguarded quality was one aspect of his personality that made him appealing; it helped him get his needs met. He made friends with the secretaries. "You have anything for me?" was a standard form of greeting. Being given something that belonged to another person meant a lot to Sam, much more than the object itself. It did not bother him that he might need to ask several times.

~

It soon became apparent to me that Sam sometimes acted restless and hyperactive because he could neither identify nor articulate his feelings. I believe that he experienced emotions as global feeling states, amorphous and chaotic. Sam might feel "good" in a general sense or have vague discomfort or feel "upset." Because he did not yet have the use of language to express these emotions, his amorphous feeling states caused inner turmoil, which gave rise to behavioral impulses for discharge of his emotions. Without this ability to identify emotions, he and I did not share the same language.

A very important concept I learned in my graduate training relates to working with people's defenses in treatment. If you want the client to give up a symptom or a defense, you must give him or her another defense to substitute for it. In this case, I was asking Sam to stop acting out with violent or agitated behavior and instead to use words. The next goal of the therapy was to teach Sam a simple vocabulary for expressing feelings. In that part of the session in which I met with Sam and his medical liaison together, I shared with her what I planned to do. I wanted to make sure that Sam would find a receptive audience for his expressions of feeling, whatever they might be. I wanted his feelings and their verbal expressions to be reinforced similarly outside of therapy.

I surmised that he would be able to connect his internal feeling state with a word-label so that we could share the same language. I began to teach Sam the words to use to indicate how he was feeling. By observing him, his facial expressions, and behavior, and by extrapolating how I might feel in a similar situation, I could guess his possible emotions. At first I gave him some choices of words to describe how he was feeling, such as "sad," "disappointed," or "hurt," but I found that it was not long before he was able to use the descriptive words spontaneously, without my prompting.

Another technique I have found useful with less capable clients with minimal expressive verbal skills is the use of "feeling faces." Four feelings, "mad," "sad," "glad," and "scared," are represented by drawings of four faces. The faces, each drawn on a paper plate, are sketched with strong lines and minimal detail to show facial expressions and are unisex. The nonverbal individual can point to the face that shows "how you are feeling now," and then we can talk about the events which prompt this emotion. Or, I may talk about an important event—a counselor's leaving the group home, for example—and ask the client to point to the pictured face that best represents how he or she is feeling about this event.

Often, in actual practice, I am doing most of the talking. This is another point at which the practice of therapy with an individual with mental retardation differs from the interviewing techniques used with a typical client. I feel strongly that I cannot ask my clients to do that which they are unable or not yet able to do—in this case, to speak cogently about his emotions and associations to prior experiences, people, and memories. Throughout their lives their deficits and inabilities have continually been pointed out to them. It would be countertherapeutic to repeat this dynamic in the therapy, so accommodations must be made. Empathic guesswork is guided by the client's verbal and facial responses. Together we connect events to feelings, behaviors to the feelings that prompted them, and memories to feelings.

Ultimately, the goal of the therapy is for clients to understand and accept themselves. This goal applies whether the individual is cognitively impaired or not. But when he or she has mental retardation, interaction occurs within a whole social ecology of support systems and their personnel, who are involved in his or her care and day-to-day life. It is helpful to keep these staff members informed about gains in the therapy. Therapy is usually scheduled for once a week and actually represents a very small part of the client's time and experience. If others know what the client is working to change, his or her efforts can be reinforced more consistently.

In Sam's case, I learned that he is a very social person. It became apparent that he is exquisitely sensitive to his human environment; he has an uncanny ability to read people's moods. This ability may be a lasting consequence of having lived for many years in large institutions for people with mental retardation. The high ratio of patients to caregivers made it advantageous for him to develop skills for making emotional contact with the staff in an effort to meet his needs.

In therapy I became aware that his agitation and irritability reflected the moods and relationships among the house staff. When staff were unhappy with their jobs or were arguing with other staff, he would act out accordingly or would report on it in my office. The staff's relationships had a direct bearing on his security and equilibrium.

~

To gain some insight into Sam's formative years, it is important to understand the culture of the large state institutions. At the time Sam was born, most physicians advised institutionalization at or soon after the birth of a child with disabilities. (Some parents refused to institutionalize their children and raised them at home; too often we clinicians call these parents "overprotective.") In the words of Roger Macnamara (1994),

> Institutional life had an odd quality of its own, an admixture of camaraderie, emergency frenzies, and stoic indifference. . . . There were staff characters and resident characters. . . . They would never grow tired of showing you their unique talents. The competition for attention among the residents was intense. If you were "a somebody" at the institution, they knew it, and you were greeted like a celebrity. Tobacco, caffeine, and attention were the unprescribed drugs of choice. (p. 241)

With this background in mind, one has to wonder what other behavioral manifestations originated in institutional living, and whether Sam's deportment represented an ongoing adjustment to deinstitutionalization and to learning new behavioral norms suitable for living in a real home. When one considers the society in which Sam was raised, his desire for coffee and soda, his tendency to grab whatever he sees, his lack of understanding of private property, and his inability to postpone gratification all take on new meaning. These behaviors were adaptations to the institutional environment and enabled him to survive there.

~

Sam is a man who is happiest when he is doing things with other people. He especially likes to go out to eat and to places in the community. He and the other housemate with verbal ability are like brothers; they alternate between scrapping with each other and being best buddies. The group home staff were sensitive to these men's need to socialize and made the effort to get them together for "double dates" with women from another home nearby. They went to each other's homes for dinner and out to the movies, chaperoned by house counselors. The woman with whom Sam was paired had an aversion to being touched, which presented a challenge to this affectionate and impulsive man. We spent several sessions talking about this. The issue for Sam evolved into how he could get his needs met.

This led me to wonder about the role of Sam's parents, usually one's primary source of love and esteem. Upon contacting them—they lived in the area—I found that they are an elderly couple who were trying to take care of each other in their apartment building for seniors. They did not have much contact with their son—limited to occasional phone calls and a gift at Christmas. It was apparent that their perception of him and his situation had changed little over the years: his father referred to Sam's group home as "the school." I requested that they invite him to visit with them for a day. Their fear was that he would not want to leave at the end of the visit and would have a tantrum. (This had actually happened and was a realistic fear on their part.) Prior to the visit, Sam and I discussed the best ways to behave to ensure that he would be invited back, while the group home staff made the arrangements. The visit went well; Sam watched television at their house and was pleased just to be with them. He did notice that his parents, especially his mother, were becoming older and more frail; this made him anxious. I helped him frame his thoughts on a greeting card that we sent to his mother. He seemed to sense their withdrawal in order to take care of themselves and feared that his source of parental interest and love could be finite. Gingerly, I introduced a discussion about his parents' increasing frailty and the fact that they would indeed die someday. In my role as a therapist, I have a responsibility to support reality and to help interpret reality, as I understand it, to the client. Often it takes time to understand the realities of a client's life. Then my task becomes one of helping the client accept and deal with this reality. In Sam's case, my job was to help him accept the inevitability of his parents' aging and eventual death but also to help him understand that he had other resources for meeting his needs. One day when we were discussing these issues I was startled when he blurted out, "I need a mother's love!" Without exaggeration or apology, he had pinpointed his greatest psychic requirement.

~

It was during this period of mentally dealing with his parents' deteriorating health and their mortality that Sam began "falling in love." Although we talked about the women he saw socially and about his co-workers, he did not feel a particular attraction to any one of his peers. Apparently he felt that their limitations were such that they could not offer him the empathic connection or depth of caring that he was seeking. His love object invariably was a warm, nurturing, middle-age, usually married, female staff member. So began what became a pattern of obsessional infatuations. When Sam fell in love, he could not sleep at night and tore his clothes. He was even more agitated, and the self-stimulating behaviors were more pronounced. He cried a great deal throughout the day, on his work shift, and of course at night.

An appointment was made for Sam to see a psychiatrist; the use of medication was considered. The psychiatrist was frustrated because she could not prescribe medication he sorely needed without first obtaining the approval of the behavior management committee, which met monthly. It was their task to ensure that the group home resident functioned in the least restrictive environment possible. The behavior management committee wanted to see extensive documentation of the negative behaviors: their frequency, what seemed to precipitate them, and what actions staff took to deal with them. They wanted to ensure that behavioral remedies were exhausted before they would approve medication. In addition, the system would not allow the psychiatrist to prescribe medication on an as-needed basis. Meanwhile, Sam was even more unkempt and agitated than usual, he was miserable, the group home was in turmoil, and the staff were exhausted and overwhelmed. After an inordinately long period, approval to prescribe medication was granted.

Sam cried in the office, his thin frame wracked with sobs. "I need love!!" he wailed. He seemed to feel his lack of love in a visceral manner; it was palpable, and I could also feel it. No amount of reasoning with him was effective. "She's married," the medical liaison said. "She already has a husband and children that she goes home to," I said. We took turns making statements in this vein; I must admit I initially neglected to take the empathic stance. "She likes you very much—as a friend," she said. I attempted to normalize the experience: "Sooner or later, this same thing happens to every guy—he loves a girl who doesn't love him in the same way."

Sam listened to our versions of his reality and filed them away for later. He was overwhelmed with the intensity of his unrequited need. In his mind, maternal love and sexual love were combined. He was absolutely correct—he did need love. What he needed most at that moment was my recognition of his need for love and his fear that he would not receive it or would not receive as much as he needs. He taught me that even a person with cognitive impairments has the ability to reflect on his life and realize what is missing. He understands acutely how his life differs from the life he would like to lead, which other people seem to have established. The existential questions he posed were difficult to answer. Why is any one of us loved? Does it have to be deserved? Must we conform or make ourselves more appealing in order to be lovable? Where were his sources of love? Could he get this need met from a professional therapist in weekly installments? Would he be loved—in loco parentis—by paid group home staff working assigned shifts?

An incident that occurred shortly before this infatuation may have contributed to his desire for safe, maternal affection. This incident, prompted in part by Sam's gregarious nature, resulted in his becoming psychologically disorganized temporarily. He became very emotional, his attention span was shorter, and some of his ideas and fears didn't make sense. Sam had made friends with his female friend's counselor. He liked to go out with other people, so one day the drivers included him in a casual get-together to buy pizza for themselves and a couple of friends. They brought the pizza back to one person's apartment and shared it for dinner. One of the drivers was mock-wrestling with his girlfriend and everyone had a good time. They brought Sam home after dinner.

Later, however, Sam began crying hysterically. He said he had been homosexually raped, which was not borne out by the exhaustive investigation that followed. He himself changed his version of events several times. In therapy, I attempted to calm Sam and understand his internal experience and why it was so different from that of everyone else who had been present. My sense was that some aspect of the occasion had evoked memories from an earlier time in his life, memories that he was unable to verbalize. It is entirely within the realm of possibility that the experience of seeing the young man wrestling with his girlfriend affected Sam powerfully. It combined sexual and aggressive elements and raised issues of power and overpowering. It is probable that it evoked previous sexual situations—homosexual and heterosexual—which he may have witnessed or experienced while institutionalized. Issues concerning the social status differential between staff and residents were also involved. However, after this pizza party, I am sure that loving a female staff member seemed to him relatively straightforward and reasonable.

Unfortunately, following the investigation, Sam's support system responded by restricting his socializing further. People who wanted to take him for an outing had to be preapproved and schedule the outing in advance. For my part, I tried to help him contain the strong affects that had been stirred up. I reassured him that he had not done anything wrong and he was not in trouble and that people still liked him. Sam benefited from this soothing, which he could not do for himself, and was able to regain his equilibrium and usual gregariousness. He pestered me to find out when he could attend classes and social clubs. I telephoned for this information in his presence to show my support for these requests.

~

Sam's current appearance is not substantially different from what it used to be, but it is no longer so prominent in my overall perception of him. More notable is his usual expansive demeanor and his friendly and affectionate nature. I continue to be impressed with the manner in which he advocates for his emotional requirements, grabbing objects and attention as he feels necessary. He challenged me to look beyond his unappealing physical appearance and to consider him as more than an accumulation of deficits, to find his strengths and to work with them. I had to modify psychotherapeutic techniques to reach his mental life in ways that he could use. First, I needed to tolerate his pacing and self-stimulating behaviors, because that motor activity was his way of discharging his pent-up feelings. Second, I was more active in sessions than I would be with other clients; I gave Sam choices of words and possible feelings, so that he could choose among them to tell me how he felt. This was one way that helped him learn to identify his feelings and to label them with words. I was also more active in the sense that I placed phone calls and wrote his sentiments on greeting cards or notes to counselors, as he could not do these things for himself. He learned from the therapy that talking out his feelings made him feel better and that it was okay for him to have these feelings. Also, he could feel effective when those around him understood his requests and their importance to him. Along the way, he instructed me in the meaning and function of behavior considered maladaptive, and I shared this information with the social support network that was so important to him. In practice this process was almost continuous, because there was so much staff turnover. Working with Sam was also very gratifying. Once his expressions of need were understood, we worked on finding resources to fill those needs.

Therapy helped Sam become a more contented person, one who is better equipped to function at home and at work. Sam is a happier person now for being able to communicate more clearly and effectively with people on whom he depends for friendship and support. Staff are able to speak to his concerns and to provide what he wants because they have an increased understanding of his psychological needs. House counselors have made changes to increase outings in the community and minimize boredom. Staff are more aware of his, and other clients', sensitivity to the moods and interactions of the counselors who work with clients. Therapy helped him to accept himself with his feelings; no longer must he believe, for example, that he is "bad" because he is "mad." With his energies freed from issues of psychic survival, Sam blossomed into the gregarious and friendly man who lived inside the unappealing exterior.

REFERENCE

Macnamara, R.D. (1994). The Mansfield training school is closed: The swamp has been finally drained. *Mental Retardation, 32,* 239–242.

16

Brad

Psychotherapy from Disability to Death

JoAnn LeMaistre

Circle of light
Cobweb of pain
Resolve of steel
Circle of light . . .

A therapist never knows what to expect when the phone rings. Typically, when a person calls with an inquiry or a request for an appointment, a brief conversation follows to verify the safety of the person calling and to get a glimpse into the reason for the call. It is interesting to note that often the form and content of this initial call are essential to the architecture of the ensuing therapy.

With regard to the case at hand, the message I received was to call a nurse in one of the local medical clinics about a referral. I did not recognize the name or the extension number, but I reasoned that one of the several doctors who routinely referred their patients with chronic physical illnesses or disabilities had suggested my name.

In actuality, the nurse located me through a local agency serving individuals with visual impairments, where I had been a client 3 years before.

The nurse asked for an appointment. So far, it was clear only that she wanted to be sure I was aesthetically acceptable—to know that she would be referring to someone who did not wear the mark of blindness too openly. Her call provoked strong reactions. I experienced her on the phone as controlling, very anxious, and critical of me. I commented on her uneasiness and suggested that her patient would need to determine whether I would frighten him. She retreated into officiousness. I had been too confrontive, in her opinion, and she could not perceive me as a potential ally for her patient. On a professional level, she was being thorough and energetic on behalf of her patient. Nevertheless, I felt that her judgmental evaluation of me seemed inappropriate and dismissive of her patient's ability to choose a therapist for himself. Why could she not trust her patient to arrive at a good decision?

I wondered why, when, and how this patient received help. Was he emotionally paralyzed and not able to act for himself? Was he just the recipient of careful advice? How is it that so much fervent energy is available on his behalf? And, presuming that I was reacting to intuited hostility, whose hostility was it? The latter is a very important question. Of the potential owners of this hostility, I had to include myself. To what degree were all these reactions a function of my defensiveness about being relatively new to disability? All my hypotheses had to stay open for a long time to come.

The meeting with the nurse went well. By her own admission, she was overinvolved with her patient. Her guilt over stepping out of the role of counselor created an aggressive quality in her initial contact. The guilt eased as she discussed her professional concerns about Brad, her 33-year-old patient with diabetes. She asked many pertinent questions, reassuring herself that I had a profound interest in the strengths of the people walking into my office, regardless of their distress.

The most useful information she provided about Brad was that he had mastered autohypnosis as a method of pain control. Self-hypnosis reflects an ability to narrow the perceptual field and concentrate intensely. It can be a powerfully freeing tool for pain and anxiety. If it happens unconsciously, it can be dangerous (e.g., the trance induced by focusing on the white line while driving at night). Autohypnosis is a skill requiring practice and consistency. These are the same skills required to gain insights in psychotherapy.

I was to learn over time how hungry Brad was for other tools of therapy, like learning to value himself for complex abilities and experiences with which he was already familiar. He had learned many complex skills in order to cope with early childhood frightening experiences. An in-depth look at these frightening experiences did not occur for months, but within the first two meetings Brad was able to tell me about his current health-related fright and his strengths and vulnerabilities as a child.

Emotional adaptation to illness occurs in stages that overlap and intertwine. Illness does not occur in a vacuum. It disrupts and often traumatizes a person within a particular life context. This context might include personal development, career development, or family and intimate relationships. If we are to understand how to help, we must understand 1) the nature and severity of the illness or disability, 2) the pre-illness strengths used to master adversity, and 3) the context from which the person was forcibly extruded by the physical limitation. The primary reliable guide to this information is, of course, the patient. In situations complicated by severe depression, other-directed rage, or severe restriction of the ability to communicate, family or close friends are invaluable resources, provided that the relationship between the ill person and the family member is a positive one. Medical information required to understand the condition of the person should be sought directly from the relevant physicians or occupational or physical therapy practitioners, whenever possible, and only secondarily from records.

As noted earlier, my initial contact was with one of Brad's nurses; consultation with his doctor further clarified what was known of Brad's diabetes and its course. Since his illness was systemic and affected a great many sites in his body, I knew that whatever mastery Brad might experience via therapy regarding his vision would need to be used repeatedly as his illness progressed.

Over the phone, Brad's voice reflected charm, a wish to sound strong when describing his depression, and an eagerness to get started. His words matched his tone. He was easy to engage in conversation and he took the first open appointment. A handsome, muscular man, he displayed a ready sense of humor—albeit gallows humor—in the waiting room as he commented on how, for "blind" people, we both seemed to get around pretty well.

The first few minutes of our session were almost too pleasant, with a persistent focus on all the good things in life. Once he was sure I was listening, the long list of losses (job, independence, faith in the future, his feelings about himself as a man, a stable sense of identity) tumbled out under the force of his agitated despair. The pain of newly lost vision brought us both to tears. Brad was experienced in knowing his own reactions. He often hesitated to speak them as clearly as he felt them, as if verbalizing his true feelings took up too much room. Once he began speaking, the depth of available feeling was impressive. Like many people, it scared Brad to hear himself be so clear and complete—

to see how many feelings were triggered by his illness. His powerful need to tell his story precisely filled the room. We met twice a week so that nothing he said would cause him undue anxiety after he left the office.

Brad was also experienced with his illness. He had been dealing with it since puberty. Initially, he had a great deal of history to provide, so that I might better understand how much and how frequently his illness affected him. Later, we looked at the darkest of his fears, stemming from the reality of the illness. No matter how close families are, or how much they are told by the patient, much of the story remains concealed. This is espcially true about those feelings that make the patient feel vulnerable. It is simply too dangerous to risk overwhelming those on whom one counts 24 hours a day.

Helplessness, when articulated clearly by a person rendered vulnerable by unavoidable circumstances, is familiar to those who have suffered blows to health. It must be recognized that those with compromised health may suffer intolerable levels of vulnerability, no matter how psychologically sound they are. If the patient is experiencing helplessness, it is useful if the therapist has a perspective in which helplessness is only one of the psychological realities. Brad, for example, was an accomplished, perceptive, socially engaged, and curious human being, who was also experiencing helplessness.

~

Therapists are less likely to feel helpless if they have done their homework. The resources and practical tools available to the patient with a disability do not compensate for the physical losses, but they can provide a means for the continuation of competence. There is a tremendous difference between the feeling of compensating for something versus being competent. One reason families and professionals may feel helpless with their patients is the failure to understand this difference.

For example, Brad was a man who took pride in doing the whole job, understanding the whole problem, and being as thorough as possible. Because his work, hobbies, and much of the way he thought about himself revolved around being able to create a finished product that excelled in its aesthetic cohesion, even the partial loss of his vision was disastrous. That he could see well enough not to run into people on the street, or to read the newspaper with effort, did not offset the damage to his need to strive and excel. By focusing this first phase of the therapy on his losses, his frustrations in the present, and how these compared to his strengths 6 months before, Brad began to substitute despair with anger. Following the shock of his visual impairment,

Brad, a previously highly social person, no longer took the social initiative. He and his wife had a wide circle of friends, some of whom were very reliable and creative in their contacts with the family during these hard months. Growing social passivity accentuated Brad's conviction that he was no longer a whole person. Only Brad believed this, and his isolation deprived him of opportunities to remain acquainted with the whole Brad.

As Brad could allow himself the restlessness of his frustration, he again found relief in the companionship of good friends. Brad was not comfortable with negative emotions. He believed in being upbeat and letting optimism guide him. He could not be upbeat about progressively losing his vision, and he was afraid friends would desert him if they knew how he suffered. By withdrawing into passivity, he was at risk of abandoning himself.

He could tell the whole story in therapy, however. He could express his feelings. Despair, disgust, and rage topped the list. The more he talked, the more he began participating in the world again. Staying with Brad on the emotional rollercoaster was hard work, not because he was difficult in any way, but because his feelings were so vivid. He was determined, astute, full of feelings and their expressions. His problems were real, unavoidable, and painful. As Brad's therapist, I had to keep a watchful eye on my own resonance and take good care of whatever feelings might be stirred up in me by Brad's account.

Aside from Brad's artistic productions, he had used his vision in a wide variety of athletic endeavors. He used to enjoy sailing, jogging, and skiing. The diabetes that was taking his vision also made it hard for him to heal, so not being injured was important. Without the safety of good vision, he had given up most athletic endeavors. However, he liked weightlifting and walking. He did these not to compensate for what he could not do, but to be able to continue doing what he could. He expressed fearful resignation that walking outdoors might need to be discontinued in the winter because often he did not feel he had enough light to travel securely. He had already tried using a flashlight but found it too weak. I asked him if he had considered using a skindiver's underwater lamp. The same center for the blind that had supplied my name to the nurse had given me the name of a man specializing in innovative technologies and adaptations for the blind. This brilliant, unsighted entrepreneur had shown me, among other things, the skindivers' lamp Brad ultimately used to continue his brisk afternoon constitutionals.

This raises an important issue for therapists involved with patients with disabilities. Sharing practical solutions or resources to ease the frustration and deprivation of physical limitation is extremely helpful. Psychotherapists should not assume that their patients are already in possession of this information. Time spent learning from occupational therapists, physical therapists, and specialists in adaptive devices, from orthotics to computer technologies, is time well spent by the therapist.

The pleasure of continuing feelings of competence is a good safety net for the grief of the terrible losses imposed by unavoidable health changes. Of great importance is the competence to describe these losses and the manner in which they are being currently handled. This, in turn, opens the door to the question of how the person would prefer to handle them.

As Brad regained a more cohesive picture of himself, solutions to some of the emotional burdens began to emerge. For example, Brad, being a very responsible man, continued providing for his family, doing home chores to ease the energy demands on his wife. Brad had no reluctance to contribute in this way, but he saw himself becoming territorial and rigid about the way in which these things should be done. He attempted to make the home run with the efficiency and flair of his prior business. He observed himself becoming increasingly intolerant of his daughter's growing independence. There were explosions of rage, accusations, and tears on all sides. He was baffled by his precipitation of so many of these. His compelling desire to replace uncertainty in the health realm with certainty and rigidity in the emotional realm seemed to be a loop from which he could not escape.

There was no one more aware than Brad of the multiple needs in a family. Likewise he knew that the impact of increased familial stress could challenge his single most fervently held value—that his health not be allowed to undermine the love and mutual supportiveness in his family. We came to understand that the responses within the family were not just reactions to the many changes and infringements on predictability wrought by illness. We saw more and more clearly that the fear accompanying Brad's sense of loss of control in so many realms had a companion terror. This terror was the fear of his own rage. We had the luxury of time to work on this issue because Brad and his wife felt therapy was beneficial and they were committed to its continuation.

During the initial phase of the therapy, the focus was very much in the present. Even though a great deal of important history was amassed, our focus was on how strengths, skills, fears, vulnerabilities, passions, and customary behavior patterns from the past were being played out in the present. During this time, much more family solidity was reflected in open communication. Brad increased his level of social contact. He seemed less psychologically taut and fragile. His smile was from within and not a mask when it was there. His tears were for all his accumulated losses. His increasing tolerance for the awareness that he was a deeply angry man permitted him to retain his self-image as someone who was self-aware, constructive, nonhostile, interdependent with others, dignified and worthy of his own respect.

~

Unfortunately, like most persons struggling with serious illness, the course of Brad's illness was unstable. Diabetically induced hemorrhages in his eyes occurred with more frequency, requiring additional laser treatments. Brad reported times of feeling increasingly unwell. An alarming number of insulin reactions were cause for more realistic worry and more frequent visits to the doctor. As another cycle of severe anxiety and dread of frightening physical changes occurred, Brad's anger mushroomed. His emotional safety zone looked as if it were crumbling.

When such crises emerge, the therapist must hold onto the knowledge of who the patient is and what coping strategies work best for him or her, because every cycle of worsening health threatens the identity of the patient. In many cases, the patient cannot hold onto the knowledge he or she is a viable psychological entity. Emotional health is a spiral in which self-awareness gained in one set of circumstances may be important again during a new phase of ill health.

When the patient's sense of self falters under the burden of repetitive physical loss, it is useful for the therapist to go back to basics. How had Brad regained an awareness of his own capacity for creative, life-affirming flexibility before? It had occurred when he first began expressing his anger. At this point that anger was much more pronounced and volatile. Brad doubted there were enough words or volume to express his feelings or gain relief from them.

To my question, "What would do it justice?" Brad replied, "A very heavy sledgehammer and the strength to destroy something massive."

"Would it make noise?"

"Lots of noise," replied Brad. And then he smiled. "The noise of a huge drum."

Brad, in his thorough manner, found a music store, a set of drums, and a teacher. The continuation of competence was another basic principle quickly coming into play. Brad liked doing things well. He was as diligent in his search for the right teacher and the dedication to his lessons as he had always been when dealing with important issues. He enjoyed accomplishment. The completion of a timed, daily practice session satisfied the criterion of accomplishment. Moreover, he was very musical, and he expanded his lessons to include composition. The feeling of creation and freedom bore some resemblance to both his artistic accomplishments and his athletic triumphs. Expression, joy, excitement, and a sense of freedom were all unleashed by pounding out his rage at the horror of what was happening to his body. His discouraging medical instability kept pace with one musical success after another. He was enjoying meeting other musicians and sought a variety of expert mentors.

~

During this same time, the country suffered a recession, and the longevity of his wife's job was threatened. A nationwide job search ensued. Among the terrifying losses that can occur to someone grappling with illness is that the insurance that made particular care available might be changed. If one is fortunate enough to remain insured, the physicians can still be excluded, along with an entire support network, by a change of health plan or location. Brad's dismay was eloquently expressed as he detailed one expected trial after another in places he could not see and of which he had no visual memory to safeguard him.

At this point Brad's kidneys began to fail in earnest. He was put on dialysis. Once again he was plunged into an unwanted reality that carried with it many more concerns for his survival than before. Trauma, despair, and emotional exhaustion flooded his feelings. The music that had been so sustaining because it gave life to his creativity now had to be sacrificed to preserve the dialysis shunt in his arm. Without the music, there would be a need to find other avenues of expression of his unique personality. Once again Brad found his direction after talking about what the drumming meant to him.

Because Brad now needed transportation to dialysis and could not do some of the things he had done at home, he had to ask for more help. His wife's job, precarious as it was, could not be interrupted as frequently as necessary for his medical needs. Brad was very clear that without the unflinching support of his wife, and her high regard for him as essential to her well-being, he would not have been able to survive. Prior to therapy Brad had diminished his wife's continuing need for him. Chronically ill patients frequently fail to recognize their profound positive impact on other people. I often confronted Brad early in therapy about his tendency to be self-diminishing. Now Brad wondered if there were other people to whom he could offer something of value. Perhaps there were others who would gain something important by his letting them help him. A close relative, estranged by ignorance of the details of each other's lives, was a possibility. Brad set himself the task of reclaiming this stunted relationship and building upon it.

~

I often wonder how much stress people can handle. The requirements of Brad's illness and the repeated assaults on his avenues of joy made me anxious. Could I be of enough help? What was enough? Could I remain open to the painful realities of his life? I was acutely aware of needing to blunt what I was hearing, in order to absorb it. This protective stance is not therapeutic neutrality, and I needed to recognize that the long-term effect of Brad's recurrent trauma on me was exagerrated by knowing I would not be continuing as Brad's therapist. My own preference for being part of the process, even when it is painful, would be substantially frustrated by the family's possible relocation. Furthermore, the conflict between completion and comfort meant there would also be relief in this change. It was another time to focus on basics and the powerful healing for Brad in the combination of expression and connection to others. Brad sustained himself when he was feeling fractured inside by keeping the others in his life a key priority. This absolute commitment to doing the best he could to protect his feelings of love for others put Brad among the fortunate few, regardless of health status, who are able-hearted. These people know their emotional priorities and strive for them consciously.

Once again, Brad's rage diminished as his efforts to revive the love in himself toward the estranged family member gathered steam. Both relatives had been caught in stubborn, stoic denial of the lack of intimacy in their relationship. Fortunately, the two family members once again lived within easy traveling distance of one another. Brad took it upon himself to begin sharing withheld information. His relative did the same. The result was strong mutual support.

The sequence producing emotional closeness was interesting. Brad knew what he wanted to do; namely, he wanted to be more open with this relative. Petty obstacles disappeared. The big obstacle was being willing to risk rejection by changing his contribution to the system of silence. Brad used to ask rhetorically why he needed to be the one to break the ice when he was feeling physically ill and had so little energy. He answered his own question, remarking that the other approach had not worked. He concluded there was little to lose. The same approach of engaging the fear and trusting this process to produce change was the same approach Brad used to become comfortable with anger.

Brad's health continued to decline. I observed in him something I have seen many times. Brad's consistent efforts to be the person he wanted to be in himself and with others meant that he was content and protected within his primary emotional relationships. Friends were active and accessible in his and his family's life. He and his wife grieved together for the many losses and fears they faced on a daily basis. His wife, an unflagging asset, became more exhausted and depressed, as fears about Brad increased. She leaned on Brad more. This helped him. He regretted all that he could not do for her, but her need for his emotional support let him remain aware of his value.

The new job offer came, requiring a relocation to a distant community. Without this move, the third phase of Brad's therapy would have been a careful termination during which his increasing faith in himself would have been strengthened. The economic necessity to leave the area harshly accelerated this process.

In spite of the many months of anticipation, including turning down opportunities in places without excellent medical facilities, the difference between planning and leaving was striking. Brad, his wife, his family, and I all had to face the impending separation. I knew the move meant that Brad's powerful inner healing, as expressed through friendship for his reclaimed relative, could not continue in the same form or with the comfort of proximity. I knew that it would be very hard to replace the medical team that had so much knowledge of the continuity of Brad's life. The new physicians, psychotherapists, and other caregivers would not have had the benefit of witnessing Brad's resilience in the face of the initial major adult losses. Nor would they understand firsthand what his early terror was like and how much effort it took to master.

I also knew that all the routine safeguards were in place. Reports and my own interest in sharing useful information would occur routinely, upon Brad's request. From the time moving became a necessity, Brad and I intermittently examined what ending this therapy would mean in his life. Months before his wife's new job was a reality, he expressed the wish to keep therapy part of his life, regardless of location. With no known termination date at first, we struggled with closure. I found this work very difficult and, at times, clumsy on my part. It is noteworthy how much the ambiguity surrounding Brad's departure eroded the ease of my staying emotionally available to Brad during his day-to-day travails.

The therapy had been productive, both because Brad worked hard and because I usually maintained a balanced position where I could use my knowledge on his behalf, let my own feelings facilitate intuition, and not be overwhelmed by Brad's physical losses. This perspective is always a challenge to maintain. Under conditions of ambiguity regarding the therapy itself, there was more strain on the balance.

We had made important progress in the therapy. Brad was not as fearful of his anger. He did not have to shut down or become constricted in his creative efforts, thereby producing depression. Even though he had far less physical energy to work with than he did when we started, a much larger percentage of his energy was available to him and not burdened with various forms of anger. As I reflected on the ground we had covered, I had to come to terms with how much this patient was someone I respected, how much I felt privileged to observe his highly creative nature, and how much like a musical composition the flow of the therapy was. If we were now in a repetition of the coda, what theme required repetition?

~

Brad was fearful of all the changes his family would need to make quickly. He was also excited by the opportunity his wife had created for them. He was proud she was being recognized for her superior gifts by others in her profession. Even so, the rage at his illness threatened to overwhelm the situation. Temporarily, he hated me because he felt he needed me to feel safe with his anger. He did not want to replace this particular therapy because circumstances dictated yet another change: He wanted a choice. Feeling angry with me made it seem that his own emotional stance, rather than fate, required leaving our therapeutic alliance. The struggles of autonomy of the self, always part of termination, did not get their full due. However, as he worked on his rage this time, as in each time before, he could feel love for others and increased compassion for himself.

At a practical level, I assembled several referrals of psychotherapists—Brad was to find the one with whom he felt best. We made an emergency plan. Given that his health was so fragile, his new doctors might know someone or recognize a name from our list to recommend.

The family wrote after moving to say they were settling in with new doctors, new friends, and new activities. I closed the file on Brad, feeling a sense of loss for this family. I also experienced an undeniable sense of relief. The knowledge that, at least until I had another patient as intense, gifted, and beleaguered by real life-and-death problems, I had time to understand the impact on me of being receptive to Brad's pain. I looked forward to having clearer thoughts based on a longitudinal view of this therapy—a difficult and essential goal.

~

Approximately a year after closing the file, one of Brad's new physicians called, concerned about Brad's level of depression. He had recommended a psychiatrist to Brad, who was refusing to see anyone. This was the result of the truncated termination. Brad was not yet finished with the therapy we had done.

I thought Brad might speak with me and that I could reinforce his doctor's recommendation. My hunch was that he had a strong wish to be protected by me now and that he was very angry I was not there. I wondered if the effort of providing the history himself in a way that portrayed his qualities of calm and concern for others was too hard when he was feeling upset and discouraged. If, as before, he felt humiliated and demeaned by his lessened physical self, his anger would be building—a dangerous situation because Brad was shutting down. People would experience him as depressed. I knew from the past how important it would be to give voice to his objections to his situation so he could move on. He needed room for his current self-definition to include outrage. Always uneasy with his anger, under the new, threatening conditions and minus all the friends who responded to him as a whole being, he was responding to himself only as someone in a strange hospital.

I thought for some time before picking up the phone. I reviewed his last sessions with me and felt the key was in his profound desire to feel connected and all the fear that brought up for him. I decided to gamble on this truth, trusting that the years of productive working together and feeling together about his accumulating physical losses would be there in the background.

Would my call be received with stony, angry silence? with massive depression? with relief? with hope? In truth, the call was met with none of these responses. It was met with a plaintive, but simple, "I don't know what to do." He sounded both physically and emotionally exhausted. I asked if it were anything like the feeling he had had when he was forced to give up his drums. The response was, "Something like that." I asked if he had the energy to listen and talk, or if I should call at a time he could specify. He did ask me to call at a different time that day, but definitely before morning, when dialysis would start again. I was glad I had remembered how important it is to ask about the physical reality. It is not just considerate; it is part of the respect for realities I cannot know and need to learn to avoid being intrusive.

In our next call, I let him know about his doctor's concern. Brad indicated that he felt defeated and out of ideas, that he was very afraid of whatever was going on physically and that the more perplexed the doctors were, the more frightened he became. Certainly these realities made sense. I wondered if this were not all tinged with his feelings of not being able to finish his relationships before moving. Specifically, I asked him if there was anything on his mind regarding our final sessions. My directness caused him to reflect. When he next spoke, the baffled, fearful voice had changed to a more assured but physically weak voice: "It is as if we could always find me during our sessions. It made me angry to be moving away. I don't want any more opportunities to establish myself with new people. I just want to know how to find myself in these circumstances."

We continued to talk, and we were reminded of different times, when being expressive had been so useful to him—whether the expression was of positive feelings or the more frightening existential questions he experienced. I asked him what it would be like to take the current emotional fear of aloneness on directly by exploring this with his physician's recommended psychiatrist. He replied, "It won't be the same. There are too many changes." I suggested the part that would be the same was his wish for the freedom to be the emotional person of his choosing, to be able to express his grievances about everything that got in the way of this freedom. The conversation continued as follows:

Brad:	"Do you think it is a good idea?"
JoAnn:	"Absolutely. I know it is a good idea for you to side with expression rather than silence; with self-aware independence rather than isolation."
Brad:	"What if they do not understand?"
JoAnn:	"Understand?"
Brad:	"The difference between my illness and me."
JoAnn:	"They may not at first. You will feel the difference more as you talk and that will be helpful to you."

I concluded by asking whether it would be helpful for me to speak with the psychiatrist. This was part of the plan we had developed before he left. His response was, "I'll let you know."

His mood was brighter, his conversation free-flowing, and he was again striving for the helm of his emotional ship. I did get a call from Brad asking me to contact his new therapist. It was clear that Brad had taken to heart the old formulation of express and connect. He soon became a volunteer in the hospital where he received his treatments. The staff had quickly recognized his gift with people. They asked him to take a peer counseling course, which he enjoyed. He found the breathing and relaxation exercises particularly useful. Having a predictable way of contributing eased Brad's declining years.

~

For persons like Brad, who have the interest and a profound use for their passions, physical illness can be a time of personal creativity. The latter does not redeem the suffering. It does not compensate for it. Creativity does not transcend by nullifying the emotional struggle. Nor does it arise from the struggle. Brad was always a highly creative man. For his continuation of competence and continued feelings of self-worth, creative expression was a necessity.

The last telephone call we ever had was one of the strangest in my life. It was 3 A.M. The answering service called to say that a confused person who sounded as if he were on drugs was insisting on talking to me. They had the caller on the line. After a quick scan of all my patients, none of whom I considered being in danger of an overdose, I took the call.

"Hello."

After a long pause came the reply, "Hello, JoAnn."

I did not recognize the voice. It sounded completely disembodied—a ghost of a voice; not drugged as much as insubstantial.

"Who is calling, please?"

"Me." Clearly, this person felt I should know who it was. I began to really worry. I could hear hospital sounds in the background. I asked again for the name of the caller.

"Brad. I needed to speak with you."

The 2 years since he left the area melted away. There was something very important to say. Only a very severe blow could account for this call. The tone of voice was unlike anything I had ever heard from anyone.

"I needed to tell you I was in the hospital." [Pause and a struggle for words.] "They amputated my arm today. I can't see my arm under the blanket."

The old question of how much someone can take came back to me. The only word inside me was "No." Over and over again my silent "No" screamed.

We talked on. He would be seeing his psychiatrist in a few hours, but the point of telling me was to remember all of who he was when we first met—to reconnect to an energy he could not find that would let him eventually comprehend the reality as a reality and not a cruel joke of fate. The search for wholeness exists, even at times when others must hold the image. Continuity was so disrupted by illness that Brad needed to reconnect with me to be reminded of his ability to draw sustenance from other people. He knew he would have a very hard time with the new physical reality. He took from our conversation what he needed—confirmation that, in spite of his (and my own) feelings of horror, there was continuity.

I saw Brad a few months later when he and his wife traveled to visit friends. The marks of the rollercoaster were upon him in the emotional tone of weariness combined with real pleasure at the meeting of the three of us. I was aware of the initial energy it took not to deny his realities and toil. I was aware of my own outrage at unkind fate. I was aware of the enduring love between this couple and aware of the respect I feel for people who "tell it like it is," and do what they can under severe adversity. Finally, I was keenly aware of the transience of human physical prowess and of how losses are eased by the continuity of feeling when one life touches another.

~

From the outset of therapy and before, Brad's journey was very hard and ended in his late thirties. Even so, Brad had arrived. I was deeply saddened by his death. Within the parameters of a therapeutic alliance we both valued, he and I had done all that we knew how to do. The therapy was guided by his strengths and we made room for his most feared internal enemy, his rage. Since there was room for all of him in the therapy, his strengths were not overshadowed by his fears. Each time he was dealt a blow, Brad needed to recognize that the rage was fear. Most of the fear was reality-based.

Yet Brad managed to help not only himself, but many others on their own roads to being as much of who they wished to be as they could. In the last 10 years of his life, Brad found love and new ways to respect himself. He continued to nurture his unique gifts with people and to use creative self-expression.

These are worthy goals for anyone's life. Brad was catapulted by his illness out of a reactive style of living into an all-out struggle to be active, rather than passive. As his illness closed off one option after another, he experienced every form of anger from protest to rage. All of them were uncomfortable to him, and potentially interpersonally problematic.

The outrage kindled both a survival response and the wish to kill himself. As his therapist, I had a chance to observe how essential it was for Brad to become the owner of these feelings, to fight for himself in ways other people would willingly fight alongside him but where he led the charge. As grateful as he was, for instance, for the personalized attention of the nurse mentioned at the outset of the chapter, he needed to see himself as entering therapy for his own very good reasons and not just because someone else felt it was a good idea. For me, helping him maintain a balance between feeling decisive and supported was an important task. When the balance was well maintained, outrage fueled his desire to continue doing everything he could possibly do. The assistance and honesty of a loving family going through very hard times together let all of them feel supported, rather than isolated. Intense rage always left him paralyzed. He was appropriately wary of his desire to lash back, destroy, or hurt. He knew he had, as we all do, the capacity to be reactively destructive. Perhaps other people sensed this and took over at times to put Brad in neutral. Once there, he was an intrapsychic volcano. Once a direction, via words, was available for some of his most primitive and frightening feelings, he was almost always able to use the energy from the anger constructively.

~

Being exposed to a patient's strongest feelings taxes a therapist's neutrality. It requires the ability to hear, listen, and attend without taking on or acting out the patient's emotions. It means being touched by, or resonating to, strong feelings, rather than being overwhelmed by them. Working with Brad kept these differences constantly in front of me. At times it was impossible not to feel overwhelmed. Therapeutic distance permitted Brad to have both his unique experience and access to the creativity that left him psychologically whole, in spite of the staggering physical losses that inexorably threatened him.

I believe it is important to realize that Brad was not a hero. He was a man, firmly embedded in an expanding social matrix, who consciously, deliberately, and unfailingly used the best solution available to him at the moment to grapple against ferocious odds. He was determined and steadfast in his willingness to be honest with himself and constructively interdependent with others. He knew when he was terrified and learned how to be aware of it without losing his sense of identity. He was committed to a therapeutic alliance in which the goal was to understand as much as possible, even though he could not change his physical realities.

In addition to being exposed to so many of Brad's talents and getting to know his wife and their family's many fine qualities, I learned more respect for the emotional dilemmas of my field. I had to be aware of my frailties, limitations, and strengths, as a helping person under conditions of ongoing trauma. I had to realize how drained and weary I became in the process. I am indebted to Brad for his permission to utilize our therapeutic experience in teaching or in professional meetings with colleagues where I feel others would benefit. Brad, a very humble man, always strove to make a difference. He made a profound difference in my ability to understand cumulative trauma and its interpersonal resolution.

Brad was absolutely right from day one. For a couple of blind folks, we saw a great deal very clearly.

17

Conclusions

Toward Farther Shores

Richard Ruth and Mary Ann Blotzer

This book does not attempt to escape its own tensions. Rather, the writers writing here strive to live in them. As we share some concluding thoughts, our goal is not to dictate an imposed interpretation to replace the readers' own emerging thoughts, feelings, and fantasies after reading these case studies. Rather, we wish to sort out some of the more meaningful aspects of these stories, and then talk about their implications for therapy and disability.

We believe that considerations about how therapy works when it is applied to people with disabilities raise some disturbing and important questions about the meaning and goals of psychotherapy.

There is no simple definition of the term *psychotherapy* as it is described in this book. Corrective emotional experiences, relationships in which unconscious patterns can be perceived and examined, teaching and learning experiences, reconstruction of forgotten experience or buried meaning, trials of new ways of thinking and behaving with constructive feedback—all seem to form a part of psychotherapy but fall short of describing the whole.

All of the therapists writing here are extraordinarily resourceful, open-minded, willing to experiment, and little bound by narrow notions of theory or proper technique. In some ways what is most surprising about the many instances of breaking classic rules described here is how routine that practice seems in context. The boundaries of conceptualization and practice are fluid, and therapists and patients/clients both seem to push against them with regularity.

At the same time much of the classic content and style of therapy applies here. Weekly (or more frequent) formal meetings; careful attention to ground-rule issues; open-ended exploration; interpretation; therapist "neutrality" (at least in its narrow technical sense); challenge to assumptions; and meticulous attention to the qualities of empathy, safety, and containing in the relationship—all figure prominently. The short-term work is not "McTherapy," and the long-term work is not simply supportive. Goals are ambitious.

Taken as a whole, these cases argue forcefully against a pessimistic notion that deep, structure-changing therapy is impossible with people with disabilities, including severe disabilities, or that such therapy must be unusually directive or focal. In some ways this statement is almost too obvious to be worth making; but it bears repetition because the counterargument, that the kind of work described here is impossible or inadvisable, is still prevalent in the mental health and rehabilitation worlds.

Therapists who are willing to be genuinely open to the patient/client's reality and to work with his or her style and level probably will not encounter many obstacles. Or, if such obstacles do present, they may lie more with the therapist than with the patient/client. Quite possibly, our horror at confronting what day-to-day reality is really like for people with disabilities leads us to externalize and project a sense of despair.

When we *do* perceive this reality, a chain of potentially transformative events is rapidly unleashed. Many of the therapists writing here find contacts with family members, service providers, and others in their patient/client's social network to flow almost organically from the more narrowly conceived therapeutic work. These collateral contacts do not take the typical forms of family therapy, in that problems are not defined as existing solely or primarily at a systems level, and they do not take the form of simple guidance or psychoeducation. Something more genuinely therapeutic is at play. When the social reality is allowed to flow more easily into the consulting room than has traditionally been the case, the therapeutic acts seem to flow more easily outward (outside the consulting room) as well. It is as if the dialectic between the individual and the social, the conscious and the unconscious, is unusually palpable and alive in these cases. These therapies are deeply engaged with the dynamics of inner life. At the same time they are actively involved with fostering changes in the world. And they do not hold back from direct expression of outrage about society, when this is appropriate, either.

Likewise, the shift from thinking about disability as a problem to thinking about how problems organize around the socially constructed experience of disability is subtle but vital. There is not much talk in these cases about curing disorders—doing things to make the patient/client less depressed or less anxious or resistant, to make the "symptom" disappear. When disabling conditions are accepted as "givens," that is, not products of emotional process, the therapist can be freed up to explore how ideas, feelings, fantasies, and experiences in the world revolve around the focal reality of disability. Possibilities of change are more ample and more dynamic.

There is no way of knowing at the beginning of these therapies what will change and what will not. At times, pain and disability in objective terms continue to be very limiting even after therapeutic "success." But, because the patient/client comes to think about the disability experience in often radically different ways, or because more underlying changes in self-concept and self-perception occur, the amount of objective change can be considerable. R.J. (Chapter 6), for example, moved from a lonely, housebound existence to full-time work and an active social life with no change at all in the reality of his injured leg and brain or of the presence of depression in his life. In other words, these are changes of consciousness, taking place in a clearly articulated social context. This makes the work more intimate than many dominant conceptualizations of therapy. It places therapists in outside roles, which is very different from more confined notions of in-the-consulting-room professional roles.

Unfortunately, this sense of great possibility is more often disquieting than exhilarating. While we firmly believe that the intensely exciting processes described here can be applied to most people with disabilities, society does not usually create space for this to happen. Perhaps we cannot make the lame walk or the blind see—at least in part, because "the lame" and "the blind" are less interested in this than the larger society may wish them to be—but we can provide the conceptual framework and the therapeutic means to transform their experience of living with disabilities in the world we all inhabit.

These cases are particularly striking because biological and psychological approaches are often intertwined. Although the therapists writing here are nonmedical, all are knowledgeable about the impact of physical conditions on the mind and emotions and about the biological processes that shape mental life itself. Incorporating the biological process into the conceptual framework governing clinical thinking and intervention is not the result of making the psychological thinking in these case studies overly simplified in any way. The deep structure of psychological thinking in these cases is closer to Anna Freud's notion (1980) of multiple, dynamically interacting lines of development than to theories that try to explain development using simpler, more linear concepts or metaphors.

This kind of deep, theoretically grounded, organized framework of thinking is something we want to underscore, in part because much modern clinical thinking is more pragmatic and atheoretical. However, it is precisely this complex governing theoretical framework that allows therapists to become attuned to the full complexity of persons with disabilities; that permits an elegant and sophisticated interweaving of conscious and unconscious, social and intrapsychic, cognitive and affective, somatic and psychological processes in these cases; and that serves to keep the work described here at a comfortable distance from more deterministic efforts. This ability to appreciate and work with complexity explains where the therapists writing here get their leverage.

~

At the same time, there is an integrative quality to much of the clinical thinking in this book. This is striking because one of the core challenges of mental health work with people with disabilities is the strain of keeping all the potentially relevant factors of the case in mind. Because this can be an insurmountable task, the many moments of failure are forthrightly described in these cases, as well as the occasions of more global failure to turn things around, as in the case of Rex (Chapter 3).

Yet even in moments of failure, what emerges is an intent to think integratively, an implicit conviction that organizing ideas (in more psychoanalytic terms, organizing *fantasies*—i.e., with associated affects and unconscious "ideas" as well) about the life and functioning of a patient/client with disabilities are possible. Perhaps this can be understood as a projection of a patient/client's desire for meaning into the therapist or as an aspect of the therapist's role as container and metabolizer of material a patient/client cannot handle. This quest for organizing ideas and fantasies between therapist and patient/client keeps hope alive. Beyond that, it works on deeper psychological levels, addressing character defenses, patterns of object relations, self-schema, and pragmatic issues of daily functioning. One can find examples of this in Sebastian's empowerment to make medical decisions (Chapter 7), don Rogelio's fight to get physical therapy (Chapter 13), and the shifts in Wendy's struggles around vocational functioning (Chapter 5).

Lest we be misunderstood, it is important to note that we often intentionally search for a "cure," a deep psychological healing. Indeed, the patients/clients in this book are very clearly in therapy because they are in distress and want to get better, and the therapists accept the contract to help make this happen. Many of the moments of grace and transformation in this book seem connected to this subtle but important communication of potential: the patients/clients do not come looking for focal relief or quick fixes, and the therapists do not hold themselves out as limited to providing that. When small, practical changes happen, they flow from this deeper level of work. Indeed, the work is generally undertaken because more narrow efforts at behavioral change or symptom relief, often very well conceived, did not work out. Although the therapists writing here work from diverse clinical perspectives, the underlying theme of the work often takes a surprisingly similar shape: a belief that the inner life of a person with a disability has meaning, individuality, and possibility; and that lasting insight about this can lead to previously unimagined changes.

~

Traditional notions of disability do not seem to reflect the realities of disability experience described in these cases. Much classic thinking describes disability as something largely static and unchanging, a deficit or a compromised function that is left after a disease or injury process has run its course. It seems safe to say that those of us writing here disagree passionately. Whether or not we ourselves are people with disabilities, this classic notion is not what we have observed as therapists deeply involved with the psychological experience of disability in our patients/clients.

Notions from the disability rights movement—that disability tends to be discrete and not multiply layered and that, because it evokes feelings, this is almost entirely because of how a prejudiced world reacts to people with disabilities—do not fit well here, either. We embrace the movement's profound respect for the individuality and self-determination of persons with disabilities and its belief that people with disabilities are a minority entitled to full civil and human rights. But we experience the psychological reality as more meaningful and more complex. We feel we have something very important to say about disability, something that the uniqueness of our experience as therapists offers.

Disability, as described in this book, is complex. Problems in one area more readily affect functioning in other areas—pain inhibits thinking; intrinsic qualities of lost functions lead to the emergence of new deficits, as in Brad's case (Chapter 16). To the extent that static disabilities are described, their static aspects often seem less central than the oscillation between good and bad days, or experiences of the disability as overwhelming at some times and more of a background issue at others. Accommodation or lack of it in society seems to change everything, from deepest personal fantasies to functional outcomes. Reactions to the disability can often affect functioning as much or more than the disability itself, as in the way core dimensions of R.J.'s (Chapter 6) daily experiences are determined more by the rejection of absent parents than by something objective about his brain or his knee.

Another important point about our work in these cases is that, once people with disability are seen and experienced as real, it is hard to see them as marginal, in either the personal or the political senses of the term. Much of society views people with disability as marginal; and being viewed as marginal, or even as invisible, changes the conscious and unconscious ideas people with disabilities hold about themselves. The anecdote about the teachers we recounted in the introduction embodies this vision of marginality; at the same time, a deep and critical appreciation of the anecdote leads to appreciating its falsity. But we can better understand what is wrong and limited in this vision of marginality from the perspective of reading these case histories.

These are common stories. They are not unapproachable. Many persons without disabilities can probably recognize aspects of their own experiences in these case studies. Many persons who do not think of themselves as persons with disabilities may revise their self-concept after reading these pages. The cross-disability view is adopted and conveyed here, made even more real through the discourse of the disability rights movement and through clinical commentary.

But there is something stronger beyond this reasoning. There is a subtext that runs through many of these case studies that talks about people with disabilities having a nonaccidental place in the world. It is not hard to imagine that R.J.'s family (Chapter 6) needed a person into whom they could project the wounded aspects of themselves they could not bear; or that Brad (Chapter 16) was responding to a very real need of contemporary society, to learn about an aspect of the natural histories of people that it does not like thinking about, when he gave his therapist permission to tell his story after he was dead.

Many of the people in this book are unemployed, underemployed, underpaid, but not beyond some relation with the dynamics of the labor market. This is not the product of a conspiracy; nor is it without a social logic. Some of the people with disabilities whose lives are discussed here do the unpaid labor to maintain households and working inhabitants of households that unwaged wives used to do (and that women still, predominantly, do unpaid). Others play the roles in their family systems, or in their fragmented communities, of receptacles of human feeling that would otherwise dissipate into the void of a work-oriented society far too estranged from human relationships. Their lives have social and political as well as personal meaning. Unlocking this meaning is tremendously complicated to do and cannot be done by therapists alone; the voices of other disciplines are also needed. Nevertheless, there are ways in these cases histories that social and political elements of experience are intentionally and thoughtfully allowed into the therapeutic dialogue; and this is some of what seems to make these therapies work.

All we can do here is tell stories that we think might be of interest, and tell them with as much heart and clarity as we can. Listening to our own stories, and to those of colleagues with whom we have been exchanging stories for several years, we find ourselves engaged and pleased by the listening, both proud and disquieted that the telling takes us so far away from where our professions began, while leaving us so distant yet from where we imagine we might one day arrive: to help people with disabilities bring their full measures of wisdom, rage, quirkiness, dreams, and potential to life.

REFERENCE

Freud, A. (1980). *The writings of Anna Freud: Volume VIII.* New York: International Universities Press.

Index

Page numbers in italics indicate main case discussions. Page numbers followed by n and f indicate notes and figures, respectively.

"True access to help means availability of all services, not just those preselected by individuals with little understanding of persons with disabilities as complex and total individuals. . . . [This book] shows how therapists can courageously accept the challenge of working with people who have disabilities."

—from the Foreword by **Milton F. Shore, Ph.D., ABPP**

Sometimes You Just Want to Feel Like a Human Being

Case Studies of Empowering Psychotherapy with People with Disabilities

By **Mary Ann Blotzer, L.C.S.W.-C., & Richard Ruth, Ph.D.,**
with invited contributors

This insightful book illustrates how individuals with disabilities of all kinds—mental retardation, autism, HIV, sensory impairment, cerebral palsy, paraplegia—draw meaning from their experiences and gain perspective on living with a disability. Expanding the traditional boundaries of psychotherapy, the authors employ an astonishing range of treatment options within a framework of fundamental psychotherapeutic principles. These skilled therapists give honest accounts of the struggles, setbacks, and successes associated with the process of psychotherapy as they introduce readers to, among others,

Amy, *a young woman with Down syndrome who electively becomes mute to withdraw from the recent loss of family members and a close friend*

Rex, *an 8-year-old with visual impairment whose aggression is affecting his life at home and school*

Brad, *a gifted photographer and musician struggling with blindness and progressive illness*

Mental health professionals, human services workers, families, and advocates will find that this compelling collection challenges them to view disability both within its social context and as a multilayered separate experience, while also serving as a catalyst for improving program design and referral practices.

Mary Ann Blotzer and **Richard Ruth** are both in private practice in Wheaton, Maryland. Dr. Ruth is also Acting Chief Psychologist of Community Psychiatric Clinic in Montgomery County, Maryland, and a faculty member of Trinity College in Washington, D.C.